CW01390428

The Simultaneous

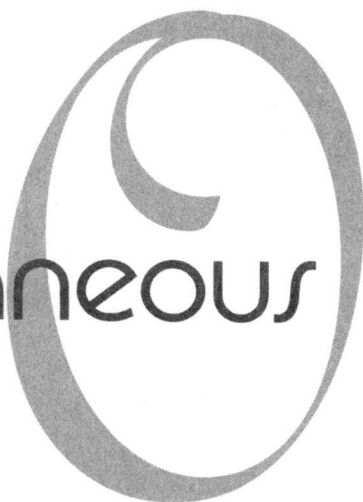

The Simultaneous O

A Couple's Guide to Achieving the Ultimate Climax

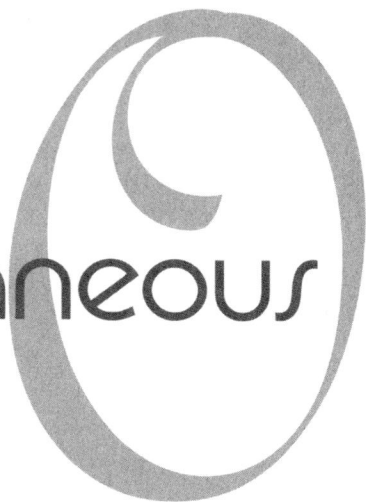

Dr. Ashleigh Turner-Corbeil

Amorata Press

*To my family. Your love and support mean
everything to me. I love you!*

Text Copyright © 2012 Ashleigh Turner-Corbeil. Concept and Design
Copyright © 2012 Ulysses Press and its licensors. All rights reserved under
International and Pan-American Copyright Conventions, including the
right to reproduce this book or portions thereof in any form whatsoever,
except for use by a reviewer in connection with a review.

Published by: AMORATA PRESS,
                 an imprint of Ulysses Press
                 P.O. Box 3440
                 Berkeley, CA 94703
                 www.amoratapress.com

ISBN13: 978-1-61243-058-4
Library of Congress Control Number: 2012947616

Printed in the United States by Bang Printing

10 9 8 7 6 5 4 3 2 1

Acquisitions Editor: Kelly Reed
Managing Editor: Claire Chun
Editor: Paula Dragosh
Proofreader: Elyce Berrigan-Dunlop
Cover design: Wade Nights
Interior design and layout: Talia Levitt
Cover photo: © sapandr/shutterstock.com

Distributed by Publishers Group West

This book has been written and published strictly for informational purposes, and in no way should it be used as a substitute for consultation with
professional therapists. All facts in this book came from scientific publica-
tions, personal interviews, published trade books, self-published materials
by experts, magazine articles, and the personal-practice experiences of the
authorities quoted or sources cited. The author and publisher are providing
you with information in this work so that you can have the knowledge and
can choose, at your own risk, to act on that knowledge.

Contents

Why Did I Write This Book?

Believe it or not, sex isn't always as easy as it looks on TV. Many people struggle to have orgasms with their partners. When people learn that I'm a clinical sexologist, they often ask me how they can achieve simultaneous orgasms with their partners. It's certainly a hot topic!

It's exciting that people are interested in enhancing their sex lives. This is how I view simultaneous orgasms: as a way to enhance sex lives, rather than a crucial factor in sexual enjoyment. In my experience as a sexologist, when couples come to talk to me about bettering their sex lives and want to experience simultaneous orgasm, they are looking to add spark to their already healthy, satisfying sex lives. I work with them to design a program that will work for them to obtain their goal.

Simultaneous orgasms are possible for couples to achieve, providing a few things are already in place. One of the most important factors is that both partners are able to achieve orgasm. This may sound simple, but there are many people in the world who have challenges in reaching orgasm, or who have never had an orgasm. If people have not yet been able to experience orgasms alone or with a partner, the first step is going to be to achieve orgasms alone. This book is designed with a focus on orgasms and builds from there, starting with understanding anatomy, physiology, the sexual response cycle of the individual, and masturbation.

Having orgasms with a partner is the next step in this journey. As couples enter into a relationship, there is often excitement and passion with sex, but not always a strong understanding of what the other person needs in order to achieve orgasm. A conversation usually needs to happen in order for the orgasms to happen. In the Communication chapter (page 20), we will work on how this conversation can happen in order for partners to start understanding each other's needs as well as their own.

Having orgasms is amazing and feels wonderful. Orgasms are often thought of as the be-all and end-all of sex. Sexologists call this "orgasm-focused" sex. Unfortunately, orgasm-focused sex often puts less emphasis on enjoying the journey. Through the program in this book, couples can learn to enjoy the journey, build upon the relationship they already have, and start having simultaneous orgasms.

One of my clients confessed to me that she was feeling a bit guilty; her partner wasn't able to give her an orgasm when they were having sex. First off, we talked about the logistics of giving an orgasm to someone versus taking control and doing what needs to be done to achieve an orgasm (don't worry—we'll talk about this in the Types of Orgasms chapter and the Anatomy and Physiology chapter on page 32). We also talked about what was going on for her. Her partner had told her that all of the other women he had slept with had been able to have orgasms during penetrative sex. I wanted to know more. How was this possible? Was he using the tips and tricks I've included in this book? Nope. He was having sex in the regular positions with no additional stimulation. Hmmm. Somewhere along the line something just wasn't matching up.

Statistics show that approximately 30 percent of women are capable of consistently achieving orgasm through penetrative sex alone. However, new research is revealing that this number might actually be as low as 6 percent. That leaves the rest of the women in the world unable to achieve orgasm just through penetration. When I brought this up to my client, I said, "Either your partner has done a great job at beating the odds, or . . . he might have encountered some women who felt it was their duty to fake it."

It's not surprising that many people, including my client and her partner, are confused about what it takes to have orgasms. Many media portrayals of orgasm present an unrealistic and unobtainable reality. One of my favorite examples of this unobtainable version of simultaneous orgasms in a movie is *Zack and Miri Make a Porno*. When Zack and Miri have sex together for the first time, they have a simultaneous orgasm in less than three minutes, with a crowd of people watching, while she lies back on a delivery crate. Hmmm. This doesn't seem to be the ideal situation for a couple to experience a simultaneous orgasm, yet this is a movie that millions of people have seen and potentially believe to be true.

The reality is that a lot of people don't know what it takes to have an orgasm during sex, and that brings us back to the situation where this terrible thought pops up: "I'm doing something wrong" or "My partner is doing something wrong." Chances are, neither of you is doing anything wrong! Also, quite often people believe that it should just "happen." Our human bodies don't always line up perfectly to allow orgasms to happen (I discuss this further in the Anatomy and Physiology chapter on page 32). Instead of leaving it to chance, I want to provide people with the opportunity to achieve orgasm together through some information and education and a helpful training manual.

Simultaneous orgasms are often thought of as the "Holy Grail" of sex achievements. Having your body explode with pleasure at the same time as your partner's orgasm is the ultimate sex rush. It leaves people feeling connected to their partners in a way that's different from any other type of connection they might have. I truly believe simultaneous orgasms are achievable for everyone, but it takes practice, time, willingness, and dedication to each other to have it be something that can be repeated, and not just an accidental experience. This book is the key to helping you reach your goal and creating the sex life you desire.

HOW TO USE THIS BOOK

Let me be the first to say that sex is about having fun. Sometimes the process itself is more fun than the end result. Orgasm doesn't need to happen every time you engage in sexual activity. For many people, sex is enjoyable for the bond it creates between the people having sex, the pleasurable sensations they feel, and the overall experience. That being said, some couples want to find what they consider the next level for them sexually, and that's what this book is about.

General sexuality books are often designed so that readers can jump back and forth to find the information that they want. This book is different: it's carefully constructed and follows a program to help people achieve the desired outcome they're looking for. I recommend first reading through the book chapter by chapter with your partner to understand what the program entails. The second time you go through it, follow the exercises and work at the pace you need to in order to reach simultaneous orgasm with your partner.

Some people might find that they can go through the exercises quickly and easily, and others might find that it takes more time. This is understandable—just go at your own speed. Start each activity at the point that is right for you and your partner and train from there. I can liken it to being an athlete: Michael Jordan wasn't born knowing how to be an amazing basketball player. He might have had the innate abilities, but he had to practice to become as good as he was. Sex is like that, too. Although we're all born with an innate ability to have sex, getting good at it requires practice, knowledge, and information. That's where this book comes in!

At the end of each chapter there are homework activities. Some require work with a partner, and some are to be done alone. This is also the way I work with people in my clinical practice. It's easy enough for me to tell you all of the great and wonderful information, and for you to read it, but without putting it into practice, it simply isn't going to become a reality for you.

I've also included other people's experiences. By hearing their stories, you'll note that many people have similar sexual questions, and although their questions might not be exactly the same as yours, hearing about them provides an experience similar to a workshop.

As you work through the book, keeping a journal may help you track your journey. Making notes of activities you liked, those you didn't like, how you felt about the homework, and things that really worked for you and your partner can help you develop a greater understanding of your own simultaneous orgasm process. This journal can be just for you, so that you are able to write your own feelings and thoughts. You can also use the journal to keep track of your homework and goals.

☽ Quiz Time

The following quiz will help you find out how much you know about sexual matters. As you go through the book, you'll learn the answers and develop the knowledge you need to become your own orgasm expert.

1. The correct name for the female organ whose   T   F
   sole purpose is to give the owner pleasure is
   the vulva.
2. The clitoris is approximately the size of the tip   T   F
   of the pinky finger.
3. The only type of orgasm a woman can have   T   F
   is clitoral.
4. Men always orgasm more easily than women.   T   F
5. Sex toys can be an amazing addition to your   T   F
   sex life.
6. Sex toys can be used with penetrative sex.   T   F
7. Everyone should be able to have simultaneous   T   F
   orgasms the first time they try for it.
8. Orgasms achieved through oral sex don't   T   F
   really count.
9. Having sex with another person is the only   T   F
   way to figure out how to have an orgasm
   by yourself.
10. The majority of women have orgasms   T   F
    through penetrative sex.

ONE • • • • • • •

Getting Started

In this chapter, we will briefly review important factors to consider on how to start using this book.

Before you embark on your simultaneous orgasm journey with your partner and work your way through this book, there are a few things to keep in mind.

CONTRACEPTION AND STIs

No sex information book is complete without a brief mention of contraception and sexually transmitted infections. Sex is amazing and fun, but it can also carry some serious, even life-threatening consequences, especially if people aren't aware of these potential risks.

Contraception

One of my colleagues begins her education sessions on contraception by asking, "What are the two reasons people have sex?" The answer reproduction and pleasure. Any time a male and female engage in sexual activity, reproduction is a possibility. Millions of people have sex without intending to reproduce, and in order to not reproduce, they might take precautions by using contraceptive products. As you embark on your journey to simultaneous orgasms, I encourage you to discuss contraception with your partner. If you decide you're not looking to reproduce, consider talking to a health care professional about contraceptive products that would be appropriate for you.

Sexually Transmitted Infections

Once upon a time, people could engage in sexual activity without worrying too much about STIs. Unfortunately, the reality today is that there are sexually transmitted infections out there that can have a lasting effect on our bodies. There are, however, also a few things that you and your partner can do to reduce the risk of STIs.

Get regular testing. Even if you don't think you're at risk, regular testing will help keep you healthy and aware of your own body. Testing is quite easy and much less scary than the movies would have you believe. The first step is to have a visual inspection, to check for any abnormal bumps or lumps. The second step for females is to have a swab of vaginal and cervical cells checked. For males, generally a urine test is done. Some men may need to have the urethra swabbed if there's any sign of infection. Finally, the last test will be a blood test to check for viral and bacterial sexually transmitted infections in the blood.

Use Condoms and Other Protective Barriers

Condoms have come a long way in the past twenty years. Many specialty condoms are available that fit comfortably and provide an excellent barrier between body fluids and skin. Although condoms don't protect against all STIs, such as those transmitted via oral sex or skin-to-skin contact, they do offer fantastic protection against many of them.

If you and your partner have not had a full STI screening done, or are nonmonogamous, or use condoms as your contraceptive method, learn how to use them properly and use them all the time! There are some great informative videos on how to use a condom properly, and I've listed some of them in the resources at the back of the book. Reminder: If you use condoms only some of the time, they're going to be effective only when you use them!

> A lot of the position information in this book is geared toward heterosexual couples. With some adaptations the information can be mostly applicable to same-sex couples.

Already Have an STI?

It's possible that after getting tested, you might find out that you have an STI. If you do, it's important to follow the advice given to you by your health care professional and finish any course of antibiotics you might have received.

Viral STIs

Some STIs stick around for longer and aren't easily treated with antibiotics. Because these are viruses, it's possible that you might have to live with them for a long time (genital warts take anywhere from a few months to a few years to clear the body completely) or forever (herpes and HIV are viruses that cause lifelong conditions). In some places, if you have certain STIs, you must disclose your STI status to your sexual partners. Even if the law doesn't require it, it's good manners and respectful to your partner to disclose your STI status so that you and your partner can make informed decisions about how to proceed and which protective methods you might employ.

FOREPLAY, OR
WHAT IS SEX ANYWAY?

People get caught up in the idea that foreplay is not "real" sex. Let me tell you here and now: All sex is real sex. By assuming that only penetrative sex is real sex, we diminish the opportunity to have sex in other ways! By relinquishing other forms of sex to "just foreplay," we lose the opportunity to enjoy these forms of sex as orgasmic and connecting.

Many couples find that through other forms of sex, besides penetrative sex, both partners can experience orgasm. But they might consider these experiences irrelevant because these experiences are not what they want, or what they were hoping for, because they want to achieve orgasmic connectivity through penetrative sex.

Instead, with this book, I want to change that way of thinking. To start with, any type of orgasm is relevant. Betty Dodson, a sexologist and pioneer in sex education focusing on pleasure, says, "An orgasm is an orgasm is an orgasm," and it's the truth! By discounting orgasmic experiences because they're not through penetrative sex, we're missing out on a lot of very pleasurable experiences! Any type of sex is a good type of sex to be having, especially when it's pleasurable. If the long-term goal of partner sex is to have simultaneous orgasms through penetrative sex, having simultaneous orgasms through other types of sex is a crucial step in the right direction and should be seen as such.

The idea behind this book is to open your mind to other experiences and to take the steps to gain the skills and knowledge necessary to have simultaneous orgasms with your partner. Believe me, you aren't going to get there if you continue to do the same things you've always done without success! Open your mind and continue on this journey, try to ban the word foreplay from your vocabulary, and, instead, embrace sex in all of its varied and wonderful forms.

Progress and Failure

When it comes right down to it, sex is all about fun and pleasure. With this information, it might be tempting to be so focused on the end product that you forget to enjoy the process. Instead, I'm going to challenge you to enjoy the process: have fun with the homework, have fun with yourself, and have fun with your partner.

As you go through this journey, allow yourself to fail, and allow yourself the pleasure of the journey. I'll repeat this mantra several times throughout the book, because it's very important to remember. Failing is OK, and forgiving yourself is equally important. Give yourself room for error, and give yourself room to enjoy! I always love the quote that sex is like pizza. Even when it's bad, it's still pretty good! Learn to laugh at yourself, and appreciate it when you can laugh with your partner. If sex becomes too serious, it takes all the pleasure out of one of the most pleasurable activities available to humans!

Setting Your Sexual Goals

Once upon a time, I was a competitive swimmer. As with most athletes, swimmers are taught from a very young age that the ability to create change starts with setting goals. This is something I've brought with me into my clinical sexology practice. With all my clients, I end the first appointment by helping them to create their sexual goals. Setting goals is an excellent way to evaluate where they currently are and where they aspire to go with their sexuality. By setting these goals, everyone has the ability to take control of their sexual future and put what they want within reach.

I ask my clients to break down their goals into chunks. Instead of creating lofty and difficult-to-obtain goals, we start with an overall goal, followed by one to three long-term goals. Once these are established, we then work on creating the short-term goals necessary to get to the long-term goals. We also look at the roadblocks, the things that will be put in their way or that they'll put in their own way to stop them from achieving their goals. I also never write their goals for them, or tell them what their goals should be; that would make them my goals, not theirs.

Each long-term goal gets three mini, or short-term, goals to go with it. Here's an example:

- **Overall goal: Own a four-bedroom home with a swimming pool and a two-car garage.**
- **Long-term goal: Buy a condo.**
- **Short-term goal: Start a savings account for a down payment.**
- **Short-term goal: Look at neighborhoods I want to live in and the cost of homes.**
- **Short-term goal: Begin evaluating my financial picture and establish mortgage options.**

You'll notice I don't use a sexual goal example. As I just mentioned, I want you to create goals for yourself and not copy the suggestions I've made. As you work your way through this book, it will become clearer what your own long- and short-term goals should be. Make notes in your journal when you come to something that speaks to you, and after going through the book the first time, write your goals, starting with your overall sexual goal, then your long-term goals and short-term goals. At the end of each chapter, you will find some general Goal Check-Ins based on the types of goals my clients have focused on. Your goals might be very different from these examples or might be more specific.

Over time, as you meet these short-term goals, you can reevaluate and set new short-term goals. You can also measure your short-term goals and feel positive as you succeed in meeting those goals.

HOMEWORK

If you continue to do the same old thing, you won't achieve your goals. You have to make changes, and one of those changes is to do homework. My recommendations may not seem like something you want to do, and that's OK. I'm not going to be nagging you to do your homework. You're an adult, and doing the homework is up to you. However, most of my clients do the homework I recommend because the overall benefits of the homework will help them achieve the goals they set for themselves.

TWO ● ● ● ● ● ● ●

Communication

Developing the ability to communicate about sex with your partner is one of the most important things that you can do for your relationship. Being able to communicate sexually is often difficult, but this chapter helps you develop the skills and gives you new ways to communicate with your partner when it comes to sex.

Without a doubt the single most important factor in whether couples can achieve a simultaneous orgasm hinges on communication. There are many different communication styles, and they can be difficult to identify. One person may feel that he or she is doing a great job of communicating, but the other person may not understand the same things or may have a difficult time communicating in the same manner. Working through this chapter together will help you identify a common communication style.

Sex is meant to be pleasurable and fun and to create a more intimate bond between people. Unfortunately, many people get so concerned about how to do it right that they lose sight of the enjoyable aspect of it. When the focus becomes too fixed on proper technique or achieving simultaneous orgasm, the serious side of sex can raise its ugly head. When people stop enjoying sex, the chances of having simultaneous orgasm are, not surprisingly, going to decrease. The more people enjoy sex, the more likely they're going to enjoy the sex they're having, which in turn increases the likelihood of mind-blowing orgasms. When people are too focused on what they're doing mechanically, rather than the pleasurable sensations they're experiencing, they're using the cognitive parts of their brain.

Communication can happen inside and outside the bedroom. I often recommend that feedback be discussed together in a nonthreatening environment, which often means discussions need to happen before or after sex. When it happens during sex, it can be all too easy to jump to the conclusion that the feedback is a negative critique.

When couples can positively discuss their sexual interactions such as their turn-ons and turn-offs, what makes them feel good and what doesn't, it makes it much easier for nonverbal interaction to be more pleasurable.

Ultimately, what it comes down to for many people is that in order to create intimacy and fabulous sex, communication needs to happen first. To succeed in having orgasms together, the communication needs to be there both verbally and nonverbally.

How do we create the grounds for communication?

When people in relationships communicate, it can start with simple discussion, or it can stem out of anger. When the communication is created organically, rather than out of anger or critique, it allows the discussion to be positive and open.

Keys to developing communication skills:

- **Remember that sex is like every other part of a relationship; from time to time adjustments need to be made to have success in the relationship.**

- **Although sex is very intimate, when you talk about it with someone who cares about you and your wants and needs, you will be met with respect and affection.**

- **Give the same respect and affection to your partner when he or she communicates with you.**

- When you approach the discussion with an open mind and a positive outlook, and with the intent to improve together, you'll have success.

- Never approach the topic of sex from a place of anger or accuse your partner of not being good at what he or she is doing.

- Communicating before, during, and after sex are all options, but each must be approached in a different way.

COMMUNICATION CONCEPTS AND SEX

One way I encourage couples to communicate is to look at why other types of relationships work.

Kinky relationships: In relationships where there are levels of power exchange, clear communication happens prior to any other sexual activity. Understanding where the limits, pleasures, and preferences are is key to both people enjoying what they're doing together. This type of transparency in the relationship builds confidence in both partners and encourages a deeper development of communication. Sometimes the communication is verbal, and other times the communication is physical.

Because there are some situations where verbal communication won't be appropriate, or won't provide a definitive answer, the nonverbal communication needs to be that much more open, and both partners need to be aware of the type of communication they'll be using.

Different physical abilities: When people have physical limitations, their verbal communication needs to be clear to facilitate their wants and needs. Something as simple as "it would feel better for me if you used more pressure" can be easily communicated verbally, whereas moving their hips might be much more difficult. By using clear and sex-positive verbal cues, communication is that much easier.

Same-sex relationships: In same-sex relationships, the definition of sex can be very different from one person to another. The openness and communication that happens in these circumstances offers the opportunity to have each relationship create its own definition of what sex means. It may be focused less on genitals and more on intimacy, passion, love, and sensation.

Older adults: Much like people with physical disabilities, older adults have to be aware of each other's comforts and discomforts and adapt their bodies appropriately. In some situations, a male partner might not be able to have a hard enough erection to have penetrative sex with his partner, but other types of sex can still be enjoyed.

By adapting and using these transparent communication strategies with your partner, you can reduce the fear associated with speaking your needs, discuss what it'll take for you to reach orgasm and what it'll take for your partner to reach orgasm, and communicate your level of arousal during sex. Having open communication gives you the first step toward simultaneous orgasms.

COMMUNICATION TROUBLESHOOTING

It can be daunting to open the communication gateway. Discussing sex is often weird for couples, as many people assume that sex is just something that's done, and not necessarily something that's talked about. Even people who are vocal in the bedroom may not be communicating specific needs.

Hurt feelings can arise when communication about sex happens, even when it's unintentional. It's very easy to feel like constructive feedback is a critique. It also stands to reason that sex, being an intimate activity, has more emotion attached to it and so any type of feedback can feel like an attack. Give each other time and space, and use good communication skills.

Use "I" statements: Speaking from a place of "I" and "we" rather than a place of "you" keeps what you're saying neutral. "I really liked this, but I think we could work on this" feels a lot less accusatory than saying "You could work on this."

Use feeling words when applicable: A lot of us have a difficult time getting out of the "I think" and into the "I feel." By starting communication with a feeling statement, for example, "I felt so satisfied after we had sex last night," it can help open up the communication on a more emotional level. If you or your partner needs help with a vocabulary of feeling words, look online. There are some great lists available that can aid in helping you express your feelings.

Stay on one topic at a time: Instead of trying to cover everything at once, stick to one topic at a time. This reduces the likelihood of "heightening" the feedback to a negative level.

Be conscious of what you're saying: Also think about what words you use, and how your partner might feel hearing those words. If you need to, make notes on what you want to talk about. This will help at first, and as you build your communication with your partner, you'll feel more comfortable talking about sex and might find you no longer need notes.

ORGASM COMMUNICATION

The first step in achieving a simultaneous orgasm is actually something people need to do alone. To reach orgasm at the same time as your partner, you first need to be aware of what it feels like and requires for you to have an orgasm. It's all fine and dandy if someone can turn on a vibrator and five minutes later have a mind-blowing orgasm, but what do those sensations feel like in the body? The following are the questions you need to ask yourself about your orgasm.

For Females

What type of stimulation do you like? Hard, fast, soft, slow, constant pressure, moving around, and so forth.

What areas of your vulva and clitoris need to be stimulated? Some women like direct clitoral stimulation right at the top of the clitoris, some like stimulation to the right side of the clitoris, others to the left side of the clitoris, some like having penetration with orgasm.

In your body, what sensations happen when you're in your plateau phase? Can you create a map of your own sexual response cycle? For most women, the first step in achieving simultaneous orgasm with their partner is finding out how to have an orgasm alone. Statistics show that women self-stimulate less frequently than men do, and there are a variety of reasons for that. In my private practice, I have encountered women who don't understand why they can't have reliable orgasms with their partner, but they've never had one alone either! Most of their orgasms have been what I consider accidental, rather than intentional. Because of the many taboos about masturbation, self-pleasuring can be a scary prospect for women. But to understand the sexual response cycle, a woman is going to have to identify how her body works in different situations—by herself and with a partner.

A woman's ability to achieve orgasm is also often heavily influenced by the cognitive part of her brain. External influences can impair her ability to achieve an orgasm. Putting too much onus on her partner to provide her with pleasure, wondering if her partner's enjoying sex, thinking about what's happening on the news, wondering what to wear to work the next day, or planning when she'll have a chance to do the grocery shopping can all affect her desire, and more specifically, her ability to achieve orgasm.

She says . . .

We've been able to come together once, and I'm ashamed to say it was when I was a little bit drunk and my inhibitions were lowered. I was free to take control, touch myself, and tell my partner what I wanted. Since then we've been close, but haven't quite matched our orgasm timing.

Suggestion:

This is the perfect opportunity for you to work on developing your communication skills with your partner. You know you've already achieved a simultaneous orgasm, so this can be a starting point to build back to what you want. Using the memory of that night can help you talk to your partner about how wonderful it was for you to take control, and enjoy yourself.

For Males

What type of stimulation do you like?

Hard, fast, soft, slow, constant pressure, deep thrusts?

What area of your penis is most sensitive?

Do you like stimulation to your testicles, perineum, or anus?

Do you notice a difference in type of orgasm with different types of stimulation?

Manual, oral, penetrative, or prostate?

In your body, what sensations happen when you're in your plateau phase?

Can you create a map of your own sexual response cycle?

It's one of life's great tricks that most men achieve orgasm much more quickly than most women do. When men and women are having pleasurable sex together, men are quite often going to achieve orgasm in approximately sixty penetrative thrusts, however long that takes. Generally, women require direct stimulation, which is not going to be adequately met in sixty thrusts from a male partner. That's where understanding your sexual response cycle becomes very important. One of my professors at the Institute for Advanced Study of Human Sexuality commented on the fact that most women wonder what's wrong with them when they can't achieve orgasm with penetrative sex alone. In fact, most penetrative sex acts between women and men are anywhere from three to thirteen minutes and do not have enough clitoral stimulation for the woman to reliably achieve orgasm each time. Most women require close to twenty minutes of stimulation to successfully orgasm. That stimulation can come in many forms, of course, but both partners need to pay attention to synchronize their sexual response cycles to figure out what exactly it is that they require for achieving orgasm.

COMMUNICATING TO ORGASM

Using verbal communication only works when both people agree that it'll work for them. Some people have a difficult time achieving orgasm or staying in a state of arousal when information starts being communicated verbally. It almost breaks the sexual concentration, so to speak.

Sex and Long-Term Partners, or Know Thy Partner

It's no secret that couples who have been together longer have a better chance of achieving simultaneous orgasms than those in short-term relationships. The knowledge of each other's bodies increases with time, as does the ability to clearly communicate, and knowing the moves that they like can help gain ground on the path to simultaneous orgasms. That being said, the only way to properly do this is to be aware of your partner's cues and not to fake anything.

Of course, this isn't to say that couples who hook up occasionally, or are in shorter-term relationships, or have just met can't have a simultaneous orgasm. It definitely happens, but it isn't that common.

Research has shown that though young couples can achieve simultaneous orgasms, as people get older, they have better control over their sexual response, and they start to understand what it takes to have orgasms for themselves, and what the timing is. In particular, men gain more control over their orgasms and have more awareness of when they're getting closer to orgasms.

Knowing your partner better, including recognizing the signs of an orgasm coming on, is part of the communication you have during sex. In the next sections, I discuss the physical and physiological signs that will help to sync your orgasms.

She says . . .

When I was younger I had trouble speaking up and asking for what I wanted. Now that I'm older, and have a partner I trust, I can tell him what I need, and he can tell me what he needs. We have an open communication style that allows us to enjoy all of the sexual pleasure we can together, and we've been able to work on our simultaneous orgasms through this open communication style. We don't always match up our timing, but it's nice to know that we can.

Suggestion:

This is a great example of how developing trust in a relationship can open the communication between partners. Asking for what you need doesn't always come easily, but as with anything, taking the first step feels like the hardest part. As you develop more open communication, you can communicate your needs in different ways and recognize that your partner may need to ask for what he or she wants or needs, too!

SUMMARY

Communicating about sex can be difficult for even the most open couples. It's a very intimate activity, and for most, it seems like an activity that we should almost naturally be good at. When we have to talk about it, we open ourselves up and become vulnerable. If we can develop a level of comfort when talking about sex with our partner, we can have a much clearer picture of how we want to achieve simultaneous orgasm.

Even if communication starts slowly at first, developing verbal and nonverbal cues to use during sex and not during sex will be one of the biggest tools you develop on your simultaneous orgasm journey.

🌀 HOMEWORK 🌀

Define sex: With your partner, have an open conversation about what sex is for you together. You might be surprised to find out what your definitions look like!

Green light, yellow light, red light: For this exercise, you can think about the types of activities you want to do, activities you might like to try, and activities you're not at all interested in trying sexually. By identifying which sexual activities you want to do together, you can have a clear definition of what you and your partner will try. This also helps couples to think outside the box and might give way to a more diverse sex life! It also helps you negotiate if there's something under the "yellow" list for both of you, and find out if those are activities you're thinking about maybe trying together.

Build-a-fantasy: It's often difficult to talk about what types of activities you want to try. By writing a fantasy story with your partner, you can take that first step, but the level of vulnerability is lower than if you were to just straight out ask for what you want. Try writing a sentence or a paragraph, and then pass the story to your partner for him or her to add the next paragraph.

This activity can be a great bonding exercise as well as a great way to open the conversation around different activities you want to try. By passing the story back and forth, you each have an active role in developing the fantasy!

Set a communication date: There are times when things need to be discussed immediately, and times where things can be left to percolate before discussion. Setting a communication date gives both people time to think about what they'd like to talk about, and by giving it a set time, it's more likely to happen than to be forgotten.

Use the communication date as a time to talk about what activities you've been enjoying and what you'd like to work on together as you aim toward your simultaneous orgasm.

Goal Check-In: Communication is often a good place to start when creating goals. When I work with clients around communication, we focus on making the positives important. Consider making it one of your goals to increase your level of communication with your partner.

THREE • • • • • •

Anatomy and Physiology

The first crucial step in getting closer to reaching simultaneous orgasms is to truly understand the body and its physiology. Many people understand the basics but never go beyond what they think they know or what they've seen before. This chapter increases awareness and helps you understand not only your partner's body but also—and more importantly—your own.

FEMALE ANATOMY

Female bodies are confusing to many people. In contrast to male sexual anatomy, the majority of a female's sexual anatomy is hidden beneath the surface, like an iceberg. When teaching sexual health education, most of the sex educators I know talk about how men generally grow up getting to know their genitals, and women generally have a disconnect.

Men start out by holding their penises when they go to the bathroom, and the jump from holding the penis when they pee to masturbation is generally not far. When men look in the mirror after a shower, their penises are kind of right in the middle of their bodies, and kind of hard to miss.

In contrast, a female's genitals are hidden, down and around a corner, and aside from using toilet paper to wipe, women can generally get away with not having too much contact with their genitals. When women look in the mirror after a shower, the labia do a pretty good job of covering the genitals.

THE VULVA—NOT YOUR MOM'S SWEDISH CAR!

When I was young, I always thought that the correct word for female genitals was vagina. Does this sound familiar to you? I think most people are mystified when they first hear the word vulva and have no idea what it means. Vulva (not to be confused with Volvo` is the correct word for the external female genitals. The vulva includes the labia, the clitoris, the vaginal opening, and the urethra. Some people also include the mons, the perineum, and the anus in the definition of the vulva.

Labia

On a female body, there are typically two sets of labia: the inner and the outer. The outer labia act as a cover, a protective layer for the genitals. The outer labia cover the clitoris and the inner labia. Although the outer labia play a role in arousal, they're not usually sensitive enough to bring a woman to orgasm.

Pleasure tip: You can experiment with sensation by holding the outer labia together and running your finger or tongue over the clitoris. The extra coverage can create a different variation from the usual sensations. This teasing sensation will have her begging for more!

The inner labia are just inside the outer labia and tend to be quite sensitive. They can vary in size and length and can change color when a woman is aroused. The colors range from pink to brown to purple. The inner labia are soft and smooth.

Pleasure tip: To warm up, using your fingers to stroke the outer, then inner labia can allow for the woman to become aroused. Going straight for the clitoris may feel uncomfortable, so starting with long, gentle strokes up and down the inner labia can be exactly what's needed to start her arousal.

The Clitoris

Once thought to be only the size of the tip of the pinky finger, we now know that the clitoris is a complex structure that's mostly internal, anywhere from six to eight inches long. Like an iceberg, we see only the tip outside the body! The clitoris is going to be one of the body parts that is important to the process of achieving simultaneous orgasms. The clitoris has approximately eight thousand nerve endings and is the only organ in the human body whose sole purpose is pleasure. That's right. It has no other job other than to make its owner feel fabulous.

The glans of the clitoris is the part we can see externally, when we're looking at a woman's vulva, and is what most people think of when they hear the word clitoris. The glans is about two to five millimeters long and very sensitive to the touch. In general, for a woman to have an orgasm, this is the part of her genitals that requires direct and constant stimulation. The clitoral hood is a piece of skin that covers and protects the sensitive glans. Sometimes the clitoral hood covers most of the glans, and other times it can be more exposed depending on how long the hood is and also on how aroused a woman is.

The clitoris's internal structure includes two legs, or crura, that extend inside the woman's body and are parallel to the labia. There are also two bulbs filled with erectile tissue, similar to that found in penises. When a woman becomes aroused, these bulbs fill with blood.

Pleasure Tip: It's important to be aware that when the bulbs become engorged with blood, the glans tends to lift up. This might seem like you're not doing something right, because the glans is playing "hide and seek," but if this happens, it's a good sign! It means keep going, because she's getting more aroused and closer to orgasm!

The Urethra

The small opening between the clitoris and the vagina is called the urethra. This opening is so small that most women don't even know it exists. The urethra is the opening that allows urine to come out of the body, and if a woman is able to ejaculate, this is where the fluid is ejaculated.

Pleasure Tip: Some women find stimulation of the urethra to be intensely pleasurable, while other women find it to be an uncomfortable tickling sensation. Using a vibrator, start with a more overall sensation and slowly draw your focus to the urethra. Be aware of the sensations and find out for yourself if it's something that tickles your fancy or just plain tickles!

The Vagina

People often mistakenly use the word vagina in reference to the female genitals. The opening to the vagina is located toward the back of the vulva. The vagina, however, is a totally different part of the female anatomy! The vagina is quite a fascinating body part and does a lot of wonderful things. It's the connective passage between the outside of the body and the cervix of the uterus. When we think of sex, we generally think of the male partner's penis being inserted into the female partner's vagina, which is the most common type of penetrative sex that heterosexual people have. The vagina is also the birthing canal, which a baby travels down when a mother gives birth.

When the vagina doesn't have something in it, its walls sit close together in a resting state. It does this through its muscular lining, which has lots of folds that stretch to accommodate whatever is inserted into it. It also doesn't have a lot of nerve endings in the upper two-thirds. This is important to know, because it helps us to know where we want to direct our efforts for pleasure.

Pleasure tip: Having extra pressure inside the vagina can feel fabulous for women as they approach orgasm. If you're using methods other than penetrative sex to achieve orgasm, consider using fingers, a dildo, or a vibrating sex toy to insert into the vagina to help her achieve a sensational orgasm!

The G-spot

There's a lot of contradictory information on the G-spot and whether it actually exists. The word itself is somewhat of a misnomer; it's not necessarily a "spot" but more of an area. When a woman is aroused, this area of tissue puffs up and feels like a sponge. When she's not aroused, this area might feel rough and almost gritty, and to her, it may even be irritating to have it touched. When aroused, a woman might find that she really likes the sensation, or she might find that it's uncomfortable for her.

There is some discussion over whether the G-spot is its own part of the anatomy or if it's part of the clitoris. For our purposes, this isn't going to affect how we approach it. Instead, you need to find out if it's a pleasurable and orgasmic sensation for the woman. For further information on the G-spot and G-spot orgasms, turn to the chapter on Types of Orgasms (page 45).

The G-spot is located approximately two or three inches above the vaginal opening on the front wall of the vagina. Using a "come here" finger motion should help locate the spot.

There are also many sex toys available to help people find the G-spot, and I discuss those in the Sex Toys chapter.

Pleasure tip: When a woman is unaroused, trying to simulate her G-spot can feel uncomfortable. Instead of going right for the G-spot, take a slow trip around her entire vulva, making slow circles with your finger, tantalizing every part of her genitals. By the time you insert a finger or toy into her vagina, she'll be turned on and ready to receive some G-spot stimulation. Tap lightly on the spongelike tissue, and slowly add more pressure as she becomes even more aroused.

The Cervix

The passage from the vagina into the uterus is known as the cervix. The cervix creates an end point for the vagina and a beginning point for the uterus. For some women, having their cervix stimulated can feel wonderful, but for other women, having their cervix stimulated results in a cramping sensation.

Pleasure tip: The relatively new discovery of the A-spot has given women a newfound reason to get to know their cervix. The A-spot is at the anterior fornix, or front wall of the vagina, between the vaginal wall and the cervix. Stimulating this area can produce a greater amount of vaginal lubrication, and if stimulated properly, women report having intense orgasms.

Glands

Women also have a number of glands in their genitals, and those parts have a most important task: to produce lubrication! The vagina is a self-lubricating organ, but it definitely requires stimulation to lubricate.

The Bartholin's glands are located at the vaginal opening, toward the back. When a woman becomes aroused, these glands release lubrication. The Skene's glands are located inside the vagina, between the front vaginal wall and the urethra. Stimulating the Skene's glands can result in increased lubrication and, in some cases, female ejaculation.

Pleasure tip: If you don't feel as if you're producing enough lubricant, or if you want more, or if you want to jump-start the process, invest in a good-quality commercial lubricant, available at most drugstores or sex shops. For more information, turn to the Sex Toys chapter (page 81).

KEGEL EXERCISES FOR EVERYONE!

Kegels are important exercises not only for health but also for orgasms.

Kegels can be used to strengthen the pubococcygeus (PC) muscle. This muscle is shaped like a hammock and stretches from the tailbone to the pubic bone. It's also known as the pelvic floor and supports the pelvic organs. By strengthening and conditioning the PC muscle, people can maintain pelvic health and experience better sex and better orgasms. I encourage all of my clients to keep up their Kegel exercises.

The first step in Kegel exercises is to identify the muscle. I've had different physiotherapists explain methods to identify the muscle. The traditional method is to stop the flow of urine mid-pee. This is not a recommended method for people who have experienced urinary tract infections, as it can result in not emptying the bladder completely. Other methods include imagining stopping the flow of urine or, for women, imagining what it would feel to pull a tampon inward to their vaginas.

Like any other exercise, Kegels can be strenuous. I recommend building up to more repetitions.

Exercise No. 1 Using the PC muscle only, contract the muscle for a slow two-count and release for a two-count.

Repeat this twenty times. Build up to three sets in a row with a thirty-second break between each round.

Exercise No. 2 Using the PC muscle only, contract and release the muscle rapidly for twenty to thirty seconds. This is called "fluttering." For many people this can be one of the more difficult exercises to start with. Try to build up to three rounds of thirty seconds.

Exercise No. 3 Using the PC muscle only, contract for a slow five-count and release for a two-count. Imagine pulling water into your body through your perineum, and when you release, squirting the water back out. Repeat this twenty times, and build up to three sets.

MALE ANATOMY

To most people, male anatomy seems a lot less complex than female anatomy. This can be true to some extent, but I think it also tends to minimize the importance of male anatomy as well as prevent people from learning about the additional aspects of male anatomy!

When most people think about male anatomy, the immediate thought is "penis and testicles, what else is there?" Well, there's a lot more to be aware of, especially when it comes to sexual pleasure and orgasms!

The Penis

The penis has three jobs to do in life. The urethra is the opening from which urine and ejaculate come from, and the penis's entire structure is involved in sexual pleasure and orgasm. The penis also has multiple components that play a large part in pleasure.

The main length of the penis is also known as the shaft. Inside the shaft there's erectile tissue, which fills with blood when a man is aroused. The erectile tissue holds blood in place, keeping the penis hard until either the man has had an orgasm or he stops being stimulated into arousal.

The head of the penis is located at the top of the shaft. The opening at the top of the head is the urethra. For most men, the head of the penis is very sensitive and contains the most nerve endings. Stimulation of the head of the penis is often very pleasurable for men.

At the bottom of the head of the penis, there's a ridge that distinguishes the glans from the rest of the shaft. For many men, this is the most sensitive part of the penis, and stimulation can bring men to orgasm very quickly.

The loose layer of skin that covers the head of the penis is called the foreskin. It's similar to the clitoral hood in females. It can be moved back and forth when men have an erection and produces very pleasurable sensations. Some men have the foreskin removed. This cosmetic operation usually occurs a few days after birth. The scar tissue from the removal of the foreskin can be quite sensitive as well, and stimulation of the scar tissue is often pleasurable for most men.

The frenulum is a piece of tissue attaching the foreskin and the penis. It's located on the underside of the penis and is very sensitive. If the foreskin is pulled on too forcefully, it can irritate the frenulum.

Pleasure tip: When stimulating the penis, explore the entire length of the penis to find out which areas are the most pleasurable, which parts are sensitive, and what type of touch is too sensitive. Using lubricant can help reduce friction and allow for a more overall pleasing sensation.

The Testicles and Scrotum

The testicles are the ball-like structures housed inside the testicular sack, or scrotum, that hang behind and below the penis. The testicles are where sperm are created. They're extremely sensitive, and care should be taken to avoid hitting or kicking the testicles. Gentle touches or tugs can be welcome sensations.

The scrotum moves up and down and regulates the temperature for the testicles, moving away from the body when the testicles become too warm and closer to the body when they become too cold. When a man becomes aroused, the testicles often move closer to the body to allow for release of sperm.

Pleasure tip: Some men enjoy having their testicles touched or even licked and sucked during oral sex. During oral sex, consider using your hands to touch the testicles, using your partner's signals as a guide to what type of sensation he would like. Grabbing or twisting the testicles can be uncomfortable and can cause damage, so use caution when playing with them.

The Prostate

Located inside the body, the prostate can be accessed through the anus. It's located between the penis and the bladder, approximately a finger length inside the anus. When the prostate is stimulated, a man can ejaculate without other simulation or in combination with penis stimulation. The prostate will feel like a firm bump. Different men enjoy different types of prostate stimulation, much like women enjoy different types of clitoral or G-spot stimulation.

Pleasure tip: When trying to find the prostate, talk to your partner about the sensations he's experiencing. If at any time he feels any discomfort or pain, try going slower with the insertion. Avoid using your nails, as this can cause tearing in the rectum. If you have long fingernails, consider using a latex or nonlatex glove to cover any sharpness. The chapter on Types of Orgasms (page 45) has additional information on anal play.

She says...

My partners have always been in control of my sexual pleasure. When I talked to a clinical sexologist for the first time, I realized that I had no idea what my own body did, let alone what it looked like. I couldn't believe what a difference it made when I got to know my own body, and how beneficial it was to know what types of things it was capable of!

Suggestion:

This is a very common experience for many of my clients. There is a disconnect between their body and the pleasure they're able to receive from a partner. By getting to know what their bodies look like, and what the parts do, they end up having a much better sexual experience, learn how to pleasure themselves, and tell partners what they need.

MEN AND WOMEN

Both men and women have two more pleasure zones to consider. The anus can be a source of great pleasure, as it is highly sensitive and erogenous. Before exploring, you should discuss with your partner if he or she is interested in having the anus stimulated. Some people might not be ready or may want to make sure they've done an adequate grooming and cleaning session before they're comfortable with any type of anal play.

The perineum, which is the connective space between the testicles and the anus in men, and the vaginal opening and the anus in women, is also very sensitive. Using a finger or fingers to touch this spot during oral sex, manual sex, or penetrative sex is often enough to create a sensation overload for your partner. For some people, this sensation is too close to tickling for them to feel pleasure from it. Others really love the sensation, and it helps them have a more intense orgasm.

SUMMARY

There's a lot to know when it comes to genitals. The more you know, the easier it is to find out what your partner does and doesn't enjoy. As you get to know your body and your partner's body better, you'll be able to identify his or her pleasure zones.

Knowing about your own body is equally important, if not more important, than knowing your partner's body. Getting to know your own parts may seem strange at first, but by understanding what you have, you'll be able to build a deeper connection with your own body and enjoy much more pleasure overall.

🍂 HOMEWORK 🍂

Anatomy Lesson: Grab a mirror! You need to find out what your genitals look like in detail to find out what you want to share with your partner. A lot of people have NO idea what their genitals look like, and from this point on, you'll no longer be one of those people!

Check out your partner: Again, just like we don't know what our own genitals look like, many people have given their partner's genitals a cursory glance, but they haven't really examined them. This can feel awkward, because, ultimately, it's an area of our bodies we usually keep quite guarded. But again, understanding what your partner has will only increase the likelihood that you'll understand what's needed to help find that simultaneous orgasm.

Goal Check-In: Knowledge about anatomy and physiology can be elusive, even when we own the parts ourselves! I encourage my clients to get to know their bodies and set goals to build a strong relationship with their anatomy. If knowledge about your body, or your partner's body, is something you like to focus on, after completing the homework exercises, make your own goal with a focus on appreciation of your anatomy.

FOUR ● ● ● ● ● ● ●

Types of Orgasms

There's more than one way to achieve orgasm, and deepening your knowledge and understanding of the various ways we can have orgasms will open up your opportunities for simultaneous orgasms! With this knowledge, you'll be able to experiment with different types of orgasms and find out what's the best combination for you and your partner.

When I was young, I believed that married couples slept in one bed, lips pressed together. As I got older, I realized that this isn't actually the truth. When I learned about orgasms, I thought that it was an easy thing that people did together, and there wasn't much thought behind it. It looked so easy and fun in movies! Now, older, more educated, and more aware, I realize that this simply isn't the truth for everyone.

Unfortunately, this myth persists today, and people, mostly men, are deceived into thinking that orgasms are easy and quick for everyone. You can see how this would create much confusion, and that believing this can give rise to beliefs of sexual dysfunction and other issues. Instead of making simultaneous orgasms a positive and fabulous thing, they've turned into this much-sought-after thing, and if they don't happen, you're somehow not as good or broken. I'd much rather see us be positive, and make this a positive sexual goal, than have it be a negative.

To get to a place where you and your partner can achieve simultaneous orgasms, we first have to understand what types of orgasms there are. If you're like most people, you might be thinking, "There's more than one?" Yes! There are many! This is great news, because it means that there are many combinations that can result in multiple orgasms for partners.

MALE ORGASMS

For most males, there are three types of orgasms they're able to achieve.

Penis Orgasm

By stimulating the penis, most males can achieve orgasm. This stimulation can be provided in many ways:

- **Manually**
- **Orally**
- **Vaginal penetration**
- **Anal penetration**
- **Other direct stimulation to the penis**

Applying any one of these methods directly to the penis can result in an orgasm for a man. Most of the time, when this happens, the man has an erection and stimulates an erect penis, but some men do enjoy stimulation to a soft penis, and that can also result in an orgasm.

Prostate Orgasm

Many men experience prostate orgasms, which can be achieved with or without an erect penis. Sometimes the stimulation to the anus and prostate results in an erect penis.

To stimulate the prostate, the most effective route is through the anus. Any time anal play starts, it's important to use lots of lubricant. Many people find that using fingers or a specifically designed prostate-stimulating sex toy is the key to figuring out how to have a prostate orgasm. Some men will find that they're more comfortable doing the stimulation themselves, and other men will be comfortable letting a partner explore and help them reach orgasm through prostate stimulation.

A Note about the Anus

Anal play can be an amazing experience for both men and women. There are a few things to be aware of and to consider before experimenting with any type of anal sex.

Use lube: All sex is better with lube. Because the anus is not a self-lubricating opening, it's essential to use a lubricant to make it possible to have anything enter the anus.

Go slow: The two anal sphincters need time to relax in order to open enough for something to be put into the anus. If anything is forced or pushed to open the sphincters, there might be damage to the tissue and the sphincter muscles. Going slow and waiting for relaxation to happen is key!

Pain means something isn't right: Some resources will say "just push past the pain." NO! If there's pain, it means something isn't right. Either there isn't enough lube or the sphincters haven't been given time to relax, or the item being inserted is too big to begin with. Take your time, go slowly, and you'll get there. This isn't a race!

Start small: Many people find that starting with a large sex toy or penis is too much, and any anticipation of pain or something being too big isn't going to allow the person to relax the anal sphincters. Try starting with a finger, a small anal toy, or anal beads.

Flared-base toys: Do not, I repeat DO NOT use a toy without a flared base! Often people are embarrassed about getting a sex toy specifically for anal sex, so they make the mistake of using anything they can find. Using a sex toy without a flared base is a quick way to land in the emergency room. Trust me: Buying a sex toy with a flared base for anal play is a lot less embarrassing than visiting the hospital to have an item not meant for anal sex removed from your rectum or lower intestine.

Referred Orgasm or Mental Orgasm

Some men are able to have an orgasm without any specific stimulation to their genitals or prostate. They may have an erection, or they may not. Having thoughts or fantasies can be enough to stimulate their bodies to orgasm. Some men might be able to have orgasms through stimulation to other parts of their bodies, most commonly their necks or their nipples.

Referred orgasms can be something that someone is born with, a sensation that triggers an orgasmic response, or a learned response.

Learned Response Orgasms

Learned response orgasm is a phenomenon that occurs in paraplegic and quadriplegic people; often when these people lose sensation in their genitals after an accident, another area of their body, such as their nipples, neck, or earlobes becomes highly erogenous. Research and information suggest that it's possible that new erogenous pathways have been created. Some able-bodied people find that they can teach themselves to have referred orgasms through repeated stimulation to another body part as they're having a genital orgasm. If someone were to stimulate another body part while they stimulate their genitals, it can result in that other body part becoming an erotic and orgasmic zone for that person. The most common area that people can do this with is their nipples: they stimulate their genitals and nipples simultaneously as they orgasm, and eventually they might be able to achieve orgasm through nipple stimulation alone.

FEMALE ORGASMS

Just like men, women can experience many different types of orgasms. Once a woman can connect to what it takes for her to achieve orgasm, it can be as easy for her to achieve orgasms as it is for men.

Unfortunately, thanks to Dr. Freud, there's been much ambivalence about the clitoral orgasm. Freud believed that clitoral orgasms were immature orgasms, and vaginal orgasms were what mature women had. Once a woman was able to submit and enjoy vaginal penetration, the sensation she once experienced through her clitoris would be transferred to her vagina. Thankfully, later scientists and researchers such as Alfred Kinsey were able to present research that cast doubt on Freud's theory, but a lot of the damage had already been done.

Today we know that women can experience orgasms in a variety of ways and none of them are "right" or "wrong," but women do report a different sensation with different types of orgasms.

Clitoral

Clitoral orgasms are probably the orgasms that people think are typical for women. The clitoris is highly sensitive, and as mentioned in the Anatomy and Physiology chapter (page 32), the only organ that has no other job other than pleasure. The clitoris can be stimulated in several ways to achieve orgasm:

- **Manual**
- **Oral**
- **Penetration (for some women)**
- **Sex toys**
- **Other direct clitoral stimulation**

The key factor for most women to achieve clitoral orgasms is to have continuous direct stimulation to the glans of the clitoris.

Vaginal

Some women are able to have vaginal orgasms through penetrative sex alone. Ultimately, these orgasms may still be clitoral orgasms and might be from vibrations through the walls
of the vagina that stimulate the crura and clitoral bulbs to
provide an orgasm.

For some women, having their cervix stimulated, either by
deep penetrative sex or with a vibrator, can feel incredibly
pleasurable. For other women, touching the cervix can result
in a painful experience and even some light cramping. If you
are interested in experimenting with cervical stimulation, I
recommend going slow and testing out the sensations to see if
they're pleasurable for you.

G-spot

Because the G-spot is located inside the vagina, it's possible
to stimulate both during manual stimulation and penetrative
stimulation.

G-spot orgasms can be elusive for some women. Often
when a woman first starts trying to have G-spot orgasms, the
sensation might feel similar to having a full bladder and having to urinate. For some women, this is enough to get them
to stop the stimulation because they don't like the feeling. For
other women, they can push past that sensation and have
the G-spot orgasm. One recommendation would be for the
woman to empty her bladder before trying to have a G-spot
orgasm. This might ease her mind in knowing that she won't
actually urinate and that the sensation is from something different and will be pleasurable.

A word about the G-spot: In April 2012 doctors identified
the physical structure of the G-spot. This news did not come
without its criticisms; although the G-spot is a wonderful
thing, not all women enjoy G-spot stimulation, and it makes

it seem as if there were an "on-off" switch for orgasms. This is something that will continue to be studied and evaluated, but one thing is for sure: every woman is entitled to her own orgasmic experience, and no one can tell her that what she's doing is right or wrong.

The A-spot

There are a few other areas of the female body that allow some women to experience pleasurable sensations. The A-spot, which is also known as the anterior fornix erogenous zone, is on the front vaginal wall, up close to the cervix. Stimulation of this spot can lead to rapid vaginal lubrication, and for some women, orgasm. This is a relatively recent discovery and still has quite a bit of uncertainty around it. But women are experiencing pleasure by stimulating the A-spot.

Stimulation of the A-spot can occur with deep vaginal penetration, but it can often be difficult to angle the penis properly without hitting the cervix, which as previously mentioned, can be very uncomfortable. Instead, try using fingers or a sex toy. The A-spot, similar to the G-spot, is best stimulated when a woman is already warmed up, otherwise it doesn't feel good. The type of stimulation recommended is similar to that of the G-spot, starting by rubbing gently at first, and adding more pressure as she becomes more aroused. Stimulation of the A-spot can also be combined with oral sex for added pleasure.

Other erogenous zones are still being discovered, and women are finding more ways to achieve orgasms for themselves. Although research may eventually prove different, I'm of the mind that if women are experiencing pleasure, then they should go with it. If they find something that works and is reliable, they can use this knowledge to help them have orgasms and potentially work with their partner to develop these new skills and synchronize their orgasms.

Learned Response or Mental Orgasms

Similar to males, females can have referred or mental orgasms as well. Some women might find that watching their partner achieve orgasm will be enough to have their body react with its own orgasm. Other women might be able to stimulate their nipples and have that result in an orgasm.

Why is this important?

Knowing what type of orgasms you can have and your partner can have gives you the initial blueprints for what types of combinations might be appropriate for you to try together to achieve simultaneous orgasms.

Why is this important to simultaneous orgasms?

When couples understand what they're working with and what type of potential there is for orgasm with their partner, they have a much better chance of having those orgasms together. When we limit the way we think of orgasms, we end up missing out on some amazing experiences. Having any type of orgasm is good, and having the ability to achieve those orgasms simultaneously with a partner is even better!

Using different parts of the body to increase the likelihood of orgasm might be just what people need to have orgasms. It also allows people to experiment, find new things they like, and try more exciting sexual activities. It should not, however, make people feel uncomfortable or diminished if they don't have the ability to orgasm every way possible.

Ultimately, there's no right or wrong kind of orgasm, and by being free to enjoy them all, you can begin to experience more pleasure. By understanding your own body and your partner's body, you open up the world of possibility to all of the different types of pleasure you can experience. Evaluating your own experience of orgasm, and what you do and don't like, gives your path to simultaneous orgasm a much easier course to follow.

Faking It

It can be tempting to fake an orgasm to allow your partner to feel positive about how he or she makes you feel sexually. It's also sometimes more comfortable to fake it rather than to tell your partner that while you're enjoying sex, you might not be getting any further along in the sexual response cycle. Unfortunately, faking it does nothing to help anyone in the long run, nor does it help any potential future partners for either person! If you're still feeling that it's necessary to fake it, you're missing out on a great opportunity to help your partner understand what you can do together to help you achieve an orgasm. Even if that isn't the main goal every time you have sex, it might be nice to talk to your partner about what you're looking for.

Although it's more difficult for men to fake it, I have heard stories about men who faked orgasms, too. This is equally wrong to do; your partner may feel like he or she was doing everything right, and really, you require different simulation or positions, or maybe you were just a bit tipsy and it didn't feel great. All are valid reasons to explain what's going on.

Sex can feel great with or without orgasms, and remembering that is a big factor when it comes to communicating with

She says...

I enjoy sex with my partner, and it always feels amazing, but I usually don't have orgasms when we have sex together, although sometimes it does happen.

Suggestion:

This is very common. Many women really enjoy having sex with their partner, but it doesn't always result in an orgasm. This isn't a problem, unless it is causing distress to you or your partner.

your partner. If you're having sex that feels great, but doesn't always result in an orgasm, that's OK and perfectly normal.

If you've already faked it to the extreme and haven't been enjoying sex, you now need to put things in reverse to get back on track. Consider sitting down with your partner before the next time you have sex and explaining what's been going on. Your partner may be disappointed to find out what he or she was doing wasn't working as well as you led him or her to believe, but overall this can be turned into a positive experience, when you work together to do the things necessary for both of you to have lots of pleasure!

Throughout this book, there are several suggestions of ways to increase the likelihood of having orgasms together. When clients come to see me, I check in with them first and ask a few questions about whether they have had an orgasm, or if they are experiencing orgasms at other times. If they have challenges with orgasm, I would encourage them to review their anatomy and find out what it takes for them to experience orgasm by themselves.

If the client is having orgasms, just not with partnered sex, I would encourage them to discuss their needs with their partner and keep working through this book to learn how to experience orgasms together.

Summary

There are many different ways for humans to experience pleasure. Some people say that it's a cruel joke that nature has played on women by putting the clitoris on the outside of their body, rather than in the vagina where it could get stimulated through penetrative sex. Instead of thinking of it like that, we would all benefit more from the realization that this can lead to a much more diverse experience of sexual pleasure and orgasm.

Evaluating your own experience of orgasm and opening up possibilities to new types of orgasms can be exciting and beneficial to your simultaneous orgasm quest. Keep your mind and body open to new experiences, and talk to your partner about the sensations you notice.

💿 HOMEWORK 💿

Identify the type of orgasms you most frequently experience: Talk with your partner about the type of orgasm he or she experiences. Talk about the intensity, how it's most easily achieved, and how the overall experience is for you.

Consider other types of orgasms: Think about other types of orgasms from the one you typically experience and whether you're interested in trying to pursue them. For example, some people are excited by the possibility of anal play, while other people don't enjoy it at all. This could be a good time to consider experimenting with anal sex, to see how it can affect your orgasms or your partner's orgasms.

Experiment with different combinations: If you can achieve orgasm more than one way, try working with your partner to achieve different types of orgasms and see how the timing varies with different types of orgasms.

Goal Check-In: I quite often talk to people who are interested in learning about how to have different types of orgasms. If this is something you or your partner is interested in, consider making this one of your goals. Knowing more about the types of orgasms your able to have increases the options for simultaneous orgasms.

FIVE ● ● ● ● ● ● ●

Sexual Response Cycle

Another key component in understanding what's happening with our bodies is to understand the sexual response cycle. Our bodies don't always automatically respond the way we think they ought to, but they do have a sexual response cycle. This chapter will help you understand what's going on in your body when you're aroused and how the steps of the sexual response cycle can help you to reach orgasm simultaneously with your partner.

This chapter also includes information on the timing of orgasms and how understanding the sexual response cycle will help coordinate the timing of each partner's orgasm.

What is the sexual response cycle?

The sexual response cycle, or SRC, is a term sexologists use to describe how humans experience their sexual desire. Women and men have different experiences of orgasm, and as we learn more about sex, we learn more about the variations that can happen in sexual response. The sexual response cycle typically has five stages: arousal and desire, excitement, plateau, orgasm, and resolution.

HISTORY OF THE SEXUAL RESPONSE CYCLE

Bill Masters and Virginia Johnson were the first to map out the SRC in 1966. They created a linear experience of orgasm that involved four stages: excitement, plateau, climax, and resolution. Their research helped pave the way for further research and understanding of human sexual response, and

He says . . .

If I can't make my girlfriend have an orgasm with sex, I feel inadequate.

Suggestion:

It's not uncommon for women to have very different sexual responses from their male partners. Instead of feeling bad, try working on your own sexual response cycle and ask her to work on hers. When you can each identify what sensations you're feeling, she might have a better idea of what type of stimulation she might need to have an orgasm.

As I discuss in later chapters, it's very normal for women to need additional stimulation to have an orgasm through penetrative sex. Other types of sex, such as manual stimulation or oral sex, are often better for stimulating the clitoris. Using vibrators during penetrative sex can also give adequate clitoral stimulation to help your female partner achieve orgasm.

Just because you might not be able to help your girlfriend achieve orgasm through penetrative sex alone doesn't mean you're doing something wrong or you're inadequate. It might just mean that she needs additional or a different type of stimulation!

has been instrumental to understanding more of the human sexual experience.

Since then, there have been several updates and additions to the SRC that more accurately reflect what people experience. Helen Singer Kaplan modified the cycle to better reflect the work she was doing with people who were experiencing sexual issues. She changed the model to include three stages: sexual desire, excitement, and orgasm.

In 1997 Beverly Whipple and Karen Brash-McGreer changed the SRC again. This time, they added another dimension: instead of having just a linear graph, they added an overlying cycle. This cycle considered the fact that women may have a different experience of sexual response than men. The cycle included seduction, sensations, submission, and reflection. This model suggested that as people reflect on their sexual experience, they may feel ready to cycle back to the beginning of their sexual response, or reflection might prepare them for the next sexual experience they have.

In 2000 Rosemary Basson came up with the most recent view of female sexual response. Instead of being linear, Basson suggests that the female sexual response is not only cyclic but also without a beginning or ending, and that women can jump in and out of the cycle at different phases.

THE CURRENT VIEW OF THE SEXUAL RESPONSE CYCLE

Men, for the most part, tend to have some variation of the linear response, with attraction and desire, excitement, plateau, orgasm, and resolution. According to Basson's model, females experience different phases of sexual response in a non-linear cycle. The female SRC includes five phases: emotional intimacy, sexual stimuli, sexual arousal, arousal and sexual desire, and emotional and physical satisfaction. Additionally, biological and physiological factors can influence the woman's experience of the SRC. At the center of the cycle is spontaneous sex drive, which is the desire for sex without other influences or considerations. For many women, spontaneous sex drive happens at the beginning of new relationships or after a long period of separation. According to Basson, a desire for an increased emotional connection can fuel a female's desire for sex, as can a spontaneous sex drive. Experiencing sexual arousal can encourage females to continue with sex; that initial sexual arousal can lead to arousal and sexual desire. Females' sexual experience isn't always orgasm focused, according to Basson, because many of the experiences in the SRC are pleasurable.

While men tend to start with the arousal phase, it is possible for them to start at different places, in certain situations. For women, it's possible to jump into this cycle at different stages; in particular, sometimes, women don't feel as though they're sexually aroused until they actually start having sex.

The SRC is going to feel slightly different in everyone's body. Here are some cues to help you identify where you are:

Arousal and Excitement

- Muscle tension increases.
- Blood flow to the genitals increases.
- Skin may become flushed, with redness on the face and torso.
- Heart rate will start to accelerate.
- In women, vaginal lubrication can begin, and the vaginal walls may begin to swell and elongate.
- In men, an erection will become more firm as blood flows to the genitals.

Plateau

- In women, the clitoris may become more sensitive.
- The uterus and cervix may tip out of the way to allow for deeper penetration.
- The labia may begin to darken as blood flow increases.
- Muscle tension will increase.
- Sensations will become more pronounced and may build as the plateau increases toward orgasm.
- Muscle spasms may begin.

Orgasm

- Involuntary muscle contractions begin.
- Blood pressure and heart rate will increase.
- At this point, some people start taking deeper breaths, while others start holding their breath.
- At the point of orgasm, there will be a sudden release of tension that can feel very powerful.
- In women, the vaginal muscles contract in a rhythmic pulsation.
- Men may ejaculate at this point.
- The testicles will pull into the body.

Resolution

- The body can return to its pre-arousal state.
- Women may not experience a resolution phase and may go back into plateau or continued orgasms with additional stimulation.

● **For men, the blood may return to the body and the penis may become flaccid.**

● **In this stage, there is often a sense of euphoria, close connection, and relaxation.**

For men, there might be a longer refractory period. Some men may take longer to regain the ability to have a firm erection, which can delay rounds two or three of sex. But men can take solace in the fact that after they have their first orgasm, the subsequent orgasms can take longer, and this can be beneficial for trying to time orgasms.

Sexual response cycles can change over time, but also from day to day. This is why it can be particularly difficult to pinpoint the moment when someone will go from plateau into climax. One reason that people get into situations where sexual concerns arise, like erectile challenges, early ejaculation, difficulty achieving orgasm, and so forth, is not being aware enough of the variety and changes in their sexual response cycle. Sometimes, sex isn't the most prominent factor on someone's mind, and being aware of that can help him or her realize that the timing might not be right for enjoying sex. Additionally, having sex when someone isn't aroused can work one of two ways: if someone isn't aroused, having sex can give him or her enough stimulation to initiate the SRC, or it can be uncomfortable, which brings concerns to mind, which inhibits the sexual response. Being aware of the SRC can help avoid the latter situation.

PORN, EROTIC MATERIAL, AND VISUAL STIMULATION

When we consider that our brain is our largest sexual organ, it stands to reason that pornographic material can be an effective stimulus. There are many ways that it can be incorporated into various stages of the sexual response cycle. While not

She says...

My partner watches porn. A lot. When I was younger, I had partners who watched porn and it really bothered me. Now, it doesn't bother me that he watches it, but that he is secretive about it. I don't know how to tell him that I don't mind, and that it might even be fun to have sex together while watching porn.

Suggestion:

Considering porn to be a sexual enhancer is something that many couples are interested in and many others are opposed to. Think of a way to approach this with your partner that is positive and encourages him to share this time with you. For some people, their porn time might be more private, and they may still need to have time alone with it, but they also might be interested in using it during sex with their partner as well. There are benefits to using porn! Keep reading to find out more.

everyone enjoys porn, some people do find that it helps them with their sexual response. Being aware that most commercially available porn is not made with realistic sexual situations, sexual response, or orgasms, and that the actors are usually covered in makeup with the lights set just right so they look perfect, is also important. Thinking of porn as entertainment, rather than sex education or a goal to aspire to, is very important. That being said, porn can help with people's sexual response.

Attraction and Desire

Porn can help couples get in the mood for sex together.

Watching porn can give couples new ideas for activities they might like to try.

63

Plateau

With porn, watching the arousal of the couples on-screen and the different types of sex they are having or different activities they are doing to each other might help couples move beyond the plateau phase of sexual response.

Climax

Some couples find it fun to try to time their orgasms with the couples on-screen.

This might act like a metronome of sorts, to help you both figure out when you should be building, plateauing, and climaxing.

This offers a nonverbal cue for timing, especially if you're familiar with the timing of the movie.

Resolution

If one partner orgasms before the other, or if both partners have orgasms, watching porn can help rev you both up for round two!

If you're uncomfortable with porn or not interested in using it, don't worry. This isn't an essential part of the work you're doing, but rather a bonus for those who are interested in using it.

THE OOPS FACTOR

One of the most common problems when trying to achieve simultaneous orgasms is that it's difficult for men to predict exactly when they'll orgasm. If they're having penetrative sex, and the woman feels as though she's close, the man may ejaculate and then, that's it. Instead of looking at this as a negative, I choose to look at it as another opportunity to try. It may feel like a failure, but instead of viewing it as a negative failure, accept that this failure is something that could happen, and it gives more reason to try again, and maybe try something a little different.

BREATHING

It might sound trite, but breathing has a huge impact on our sexual response cycle. Learning how to breathe together can help couples not only match rhythms but also sync their movements, their SRC, and their orgasms.

Method No. 1

- Sit together with your partner in a quiet place.
- Face each other, sitting in a comfortable position.
- Hold hands and look at each other to center yourselves.
- Identify who will be the leader; as that person inhales, mirror his or her breathing.
- Try to breathe as naturally as possible.
- Maintain this for five minutes, or longer if possible.
- Switch who's leading and repeat.

Method No. 2

- Lie down on the floor in a comfortable position next to your partner.
- Place your hand on your partner's upper abdomen and have him or her do the same to you.
- Identify who will be the leader; as that person inhales, mirror his or her breathing.

- Try to breathe as naturally as possible.
- Maintain this for five minutes, or longer if possible.
- Switch who's leading and repeat.

Method No. 3

- Lie down in a spoon position (on your sides, lying together lengthwise with one person's chest on the other person's back).
- Let the person in the front lead the breathing.
- Use your body to sense his or her breath.
- Try to breathe as naturally as possible.
- Maintain this for five minutes, or longer if possible.
- Switch positions, and let the other partner lead.

SEX DRIVE AND SENSATIONS

One sex educator I've worked with has the most fabulous way of encapsulating the human sex drive. She discusses it through the five senses. Each sense plays a big role in our arousal and desire to have sex. For women and men who are concerned about increasing their sex drive, using the five senses can help stimulate their desire.

Sensate focus is something that speaks to these sensations and how they feel within the body. Instead of focusing on the orgasm, focus on the smell, taste, sound, touch, and sights that you're experiencing. The awareness of these sensations can help you stay in the moment and enjoy the experience as well as connect you more closely to your partner.

Smell

There's ample research on smells and pheromones and how they can affect attraction and sexual desire. For some people, the smell of their partner's sweat can be enough to send them straight into the sexual response cycle. Others prefer delicate smells like vanilla, cucumber, lavender, and certain foods like apples or strawberries to help them get into the mood. As scent and memory are strongly connected, a certain scent might remind people of something. A pleasing scent can create a positive environment, and using scented candles can help set the scene. The subtle shift of scent can change the way we think about the room and sets the stage for sex to happen.

Research into the connection between smell and sex suggests that there are certain scents that actually increase the blood flow to the genitals. Although there is inconclusive evidence as to why this occurs, it has been suggested that it could be as simple as the scent creating a feeling of happiness and relaxation, which provides people the ability to enjoy themselves.

Taste

There are certain tastes and foods that people find make them feel sexier. For many people, the connection between food and sex could be similar to smell in that certain tastes encourage happiness and relaxation, which can result in people feeling sexier and more comfortable. Strawberries and champagne, oysters, chocolate, and honey can all be tastes that make people feel sexy. Some people find that they might really enjoy foods and tastes that remind them of certain nights or dates. People might also want to incorporate these tastes into their sex play.

Although most research suggests that there is not a specific connection between certain tastes and sex, there are foods that elicit physiological responses in the body that can be beneficial to sex, such as increased blood flow, heightened nerve sensitivity, and increase in certain hormonal responses. Some foods that can encourage these types of responses include oysters, red wine, bananas, chocolate, spicy peppers, and avocados.

Sound

Setting the mood for many people includes having a certain type of sound playing. Depending on what they like, they might try to find a beat that helps keep them in rhythm, or they might try to find more of an ambient sound that creates consistent and fluid sounds. Others may prefer some soulful jazz. Most people are not interested in Top 40 music during sex, as it can be distracting.

Touch

Needless to say, touch plays a big role in sexual response. But there's a huge variation on touch and how it can be used to increase the sexual response and build sexual tension to help someone get from the arousal stage to the plateau stage easily. Using different types of fabrics, feathers, and other different tactile sensations gently, or more firmly, across the skin can titillate people and create heightened arousal. Different types of touch—soft, gentle, firm, hard, and so forth—can also affect someone's sexual response.

Massage can also help put someone in the mood for sex and often is used as a precursor to different sexual activities.

Many different places of the body can be receptive to these different types and aspects of touch. Everyone has a slightly different request for the type of touch they'd like to experience, and some types of touch might not be what they expect to enjoy.

Sight

Similar to touch, sight can play a big role in the sexual response cycle. From watching porn to glancing at your partner's sexy body, to watching the sexual orgasms meld together with penetration, visuals can help stimulate the mental aspect of the sexual response cycle.

Setting the scene with softer lighting can also make both partners feel sexier and less like they're under the harsh glare of fluorescent lights. It also gives a nice alternative to having sex in the pitch black. For people who are self-conscious, having softer lighting can create a more comfortable feeling for them, helping them feel less aware of their flaws.

Another fascinating aspect of sight is to take away sight altogether. Using a blindfold minimizes the sense of sight while maximizing the other senses.

As you go through the book, you'll notice different activities that fit into different aspects of these senses and the sex drive.

SUMMARY

The sexual response cycle is an integral part of getting to simultaneous orgasms. Understanding our own bodies and how they respond to sexual stimuli is a piece that most of us miss out on when we think about our orgasms. Orgasms feel great, but without the comprehension of how they happen in our own bodies, we can't make our own sexual response maps.

When we want to synchronize our orgasms with our partner's orgasms, we have to understand not only our own cycle but also our partner's cycle. Having a connection through breathing can help enhance the connection between partners. Synchronizing breathing often helps us become more in tune with what we're experiencing as well as with what our partner is experiencing.

Finally, setting the scene properly can have an effect on our experience of the sex drive and sexual response. Try using your senses to speed up or slow down your sexual response. Set the scene to make it visually appealing for you and your partner. Add scents that make you and your partner feel sexy, and bring some food and wine into the bedroom. Consider using soft fabrics to massage your partner, or buy a new set of soft sheets. Play soft music or gentle nature sounds to create a relaxing environment.

✿ HOMEWORK ✿

Your very own SRC: As I've discussed, sexual response cycles don't always happen in a linear fashion. Learning about your own SRC, and figuring out exactly what it takes for you to achieve orgasm, creates a foundation for the simultaneous orgasm. Using the information on sexual response, create your own chart of what your sexual response looks like. Do this a few times (women especially) and notice how things change during the menstrual cycle and how emotions, stress, different senses, and breathing can affect your cycle.

Practice breathing with your partner: Follow the cycle of breathing from this chapter. Work with your partner and experiment with breathing when you're having sex together. Start by identifying when your partner's breathing changes and when yours changes.

Practice sensate focus: Working with your partner, create the sensate focus connection through intimate activities. Hand massage is generally an excellent sensate focus activity. People find that by developing an awareness of how their partner is touching them, they can connect on a deeper level. Identify how you and your partner can excite your sex drive with your senses. Using the five senses, play with different sex drive factors and see how changing things can affect your sexual response. Try working with your partner to set different scenes to heighten your sex drive.

Goal Check-In: The SRC is often a challenge to fully understand, as it frequently changes from person to person, and even daily for an individual. Male clients often have questions about delaying ejaculation and how they can gain more control over their orgasm. If this is a goal you are interested in working toward, consider starting with understanding your own SRC, and how your body responds to different types of stimuli.

SIX ● ● ● ● ● ● ●

Self-Pleasuring

Not only is masturbation an amazing way to get to know your own body and your sexual response cycle, it can also be an excellent way to connect with your partner. Because masturbation is still taboo, it can help forge a connection between partners, allowing them to discuss and experience masturbation together. As you'll see, mutual stimulation can be the first breakthrough you'll have in trying to achieve simultaneous orgasm.

The single most important thing that you can do for yourself sexually is to understand your own body. When it comes to pleasure and orgasms, knowing your body is the key to identifying exactly what it takes to achieve your own orgasm, and also what you need to communicate to your partner in terms of your wants and needs.

I can't begin to tell you the number of men I've heard say, "Hand jobs are OK, but I do it better myself." Yet when I ask if they've ever explained to their partners what they want, most of them say no. Masturbation is potentially one of the final frontiers for comfortable sexual discussion. Women talk to their friends about sex, but generally not about masturbation. Men talk to their friends about sex, but almost never about masturbation. Sex toys have changed things a little for women, and thanks to *Sex and the City*, most folks know at least a little bit about the Rabbit vibrator. The Rabbit opened the door for some discussion around vibrator usage and masturbation, but it's still a topic that rarely gets brought up. In relationships, it tends to be the least discussed sexual topic around.

This is so unfortunate, because self-pleasuring is such an amazingly useful tool when it comes to timing orgasms with partners. Understanding what types of touches it takes to bring your partner to a place of orgasm can be found out through self-pleasuring and mutual self-pleasuring. As the aforementioned men in my example show, we know our own bodies the best, and by communicating what we like to our partners, they will have a clearer understanding of what we like, and as a result the sex is going to be that much more amazing and that much more orgasmic.

There's no right or wrong way to self-pleasure. The way that you enjoy your own pleasure is the way that you do it, and because everyone's bodies are so unique, you might find that your method is different from everyone else you know!

GETTING TO KNOW YOU

When I work with clients, I talk about masturbation and self-pleasuring. Most people have heard the word masturbation and have a good sense of what that means. I try to rephrase the act of stimulating yourself to orgasm with a term I learned at grad school: self-pleasuring. Masturbation is a term derived from Latin, literally meaning, "to disturb with the hand." Although the change is subtle, the term "self-pleasuring" is much more sex-positive and offers a much more positive connotation of what it actually is that we're doing when we're stimulating ourselves.

Self-pleasuring can also mean a variety of things; taking a bath and relaxing, for example, can be self-pleasuring and a self-love activity. Self-pleasuring can also mean taking the time to stimulate your own body to pleasure, a much more pleasant image than "disturbing with the hand."

Having orgasms through masturbation is generally the way people achieve their first orgasms, especially for most men. Waiting for someone else to give you an orgasm isn't going to be effective; when we don't know what it takes for our own bodies to have an orgasm, we aren't going to be prepared to have one with our partners. In fact, I try to change the language of my clients when they say that their partner "gave" them an orgasm. Instead, think of it as your body being given pleasure, achieving orgasm, or having an orgasm.

Self-pleasuring can be much more than just getting off. A lot of the time, people use a "get in, get off, get out" mentality. Instead of doing this, consider spending more time, rather than less, and not setting a specific goal. Orgasms are wonderful, but because of the orgasm-centric way of thinking about

She says . . .

I feel bad when I can't have an orgasm because I know my boyfriend feels bad, like he's not doing enough to give me an orgasm.

Suggestion:

This is a tricky situation. When people are concerned that they aren't doing enough, it's because they aren't. But it's not out of lack of care—it's usually out of lack of information and knowledge. In this situation, I recommend starting with mutual masturbation and talking to your partner about what types of stimulation you're missing out on.

Also, sometimes, you have to take control for yourself. If you're waiting for him to "give" you an orgasm, it might never happen! Be an active participant in your own sex life and communicate your needs. Give your partner the knowledge he or she needs to stimulate your body to orgasm.

sex, we often miss out on the pleasure that can be associated with getting to the orgasm!

Learning how to discuss self-pleasuring helps normalize the process. Although it's an activity that most people do alone the majority of the time, we also cook, clean, bathe, shop, eat, watch TV, and work alone most of our adult lives, but we still find ways to talk about these things. Self-pleasuring is not really all that different when you think about it! It's just that because it has to do with sex and pleasure, it somehow is a less appropriate conversation topic. When I start talking about this in workshops, people generally open up quickly and start talking about their own experiences. It's refreshing to see people become comfortable almost instantly, because they realize that it's a safe space to talk self-pleasuring.

FEMALES AND MASTURBATION/ SELF-PLEASURING

Many times, female clients will come in for a session because they have never experienced an orgasm. In the first session assessment, I often will find out that this woman doesn't masturbate. Somehow, one way or another, they learned that masturbation was either unnecessary, dirty, wrong, or something that only naughty women did. Others never felt the need or desire to do it and expected that their partners would be responsible for their orgasms. Without masturbating, these women have never had the opportunity to identify what the sensations building up to an orgasm feel like and often don't know what it would take for them to have an orgasm. I encourage them to masturbate in order to start to understand the types of touch and sensation they like, and to understand how the sexual response feels in their body. Without masturbation, many of these women will never experience orgasms.

For women, there are a few things to keep in mind with orgasms and self-pleasuring.

Find out what feels good and what type of stimulation you like. Some women like having pressure in their vaginas as they stimulate the clitoris. Some women like this pressure to be constant, without movement, while other women like the stimulation to be more of an in-and-out sensation.

Loosen up the hips!

Try relaxing the muscles and then tensing the muscles.

Breathing can make all the difference. Some women find that deep breaths might become shallower as they get close, while other women find that they take deeper breaths as they get closer to orgasm. Again, some women find that as they get very close to climax they might hold their breath, while for other women that detracts from the orgasm, or even prevents them from tipping over the edge to orgasm.

Don't imagine your orgasm is going to be anything like the orgasms that happen in porn. Try using your hand to stimulate the clitoris. Try a vibrator to stimulate the clitoris. Experiment with finding your G-spot. For more suggestions for females trying to achieve orgasms, turn to the Troubleshooting chapter (page 128).

How is this applicable to simultaneous orgasms?

One of the first steps to simultaneous orgasms is, of course, being orgasmic when alone and learning what it takes to be orgasmic alone. For some people the next step is to get comfortable being orgasmic with, or in front of, their partners. Many factors can contribute to why this might be difficult, but the most common reasons are shame or embarrassment, worry about appearance, and inability to relinquish control with or to a partner.

When situations like this arise, we have to work backward and figure out how big a block this is and how far away the significant other needs to be in order for the other person to have an orgasm. We start with the partner out of the house, and once that's OK, then we have them in the other room. Once that's OK, we bring them closer, so that they can be in the room but not on the bed or within touching distance. For most people, this is where the challenge arises, and it takes time to get past this. Once people can achieve and orgasm reliably with their partner in the room, I encourage both partners to hold or caress each other as they stimulate themselves to orgasm. For some people, this progression can take time, but ultimately, it helps them move to the place they're trying to get to.

Another option, if both partners are comfortable with this, is using a blindfold. By taking away the visual, the partner experiencing difficulty can create their own fantasy situation, while their partner silently watches.

SELF-PLEASURING TOGETHER

When both partners feel comfortable with self-pleasuring, they can discuss the potential for self-pleasuring together. Watching your partner stimulate himself or herself is very intimate, and maybe even more intimate than penetrative sex. The taboo of self-pleasuring helps elevate this type of sex to a highly erotic activity. To add an extra level, sit across the room from each other so you can't touch each other, even if you want to! The "hands off" aspect of this move creates more tension and allows for a better vantage point to enjoy the view. It's almost like watching your own personal erotic movie.

This can also help your partner identify what types of touches you like with manual stimulation.

When self-pleasuring together, it's important to recognize that you might be able to reach simultaneous orgasms together, but without touching each other. This is OK, as it's a first step in experiencing orgasm at the same time.

MUTUAL SELF-PLEASURING, OR MANUAL STIMULATION

Mutual self-pleasuring can be a delicious experience to share with your partner. Getting to know his or her body better is the next crucial step toward simultaneous orgasms!

When couples get comfortable with their own self-pleasuring experience, they can try mutual self-pleasuring, where each partner stimulates the other person's genitals by hand. For some people, this might feel like a flashback to high school, when they first started experimenting sexually, but this is a great way to have simultaneous orgasms! Because we're used to doing a lot with our fingers and our hands, we're able to have great precision when using them for sex. Our fingers have more dexterity than our genitals and can be more accurate than we can be with our bodies or genitals.

Set aside some time to enjoy mutual stimulation, and allow yourselves to explore the different sensations you feel using digital touch. For some, this can be a weird sensation; you might be used to having only penetrative sex, and this might feel more personal. For others, this type of stimulation might feel better than sex!

Work with your partner to discover the types of sensations you like: what you want more of and what you want less of. This is also a good opportunity to practice communicating these desires to each other.

SUMMARY

Self-pleasuring is underrated and often has that negative connotation attached to it. In reality, it's something you can do for yourself and something you can share with your partner. Understanding your own pleasure and your own body will help build toward the orgasms you hope to share with your partner.

Without knowing how to achieve orgasm by ourselves, we can only hope that our partners will figure out the magic formula it takes to have orgasms. Thinking of our partner "giving" us an orgasm isn't going to help us achieve simultaneous orgasms; instead, it puts us into a passive role where we're no longer actively participating.

By sharing mutual stimulation situations with your partner, you create awareness around communication and your own pleasure that will give you the foundation you need to move forward. This foundation will help guide you together as you work on your sexual responses, timing, and enjoyment. In this stage of your journey, remember to be receptive to feedback from your partner, who knows his or her own body better than anyone else, and the information your partner gives you about himself or herself will be invaluable!

Don't discredit any simultaneous orgasms you're able to achieve this way. They still count, and they're still simultaneous. It's in this stage of the journey that you truly begin to understand each other's needs and sexual response cycles!

☞ HOMEWORK ☜

Map your orgasm: A lot of people assume that everyone gets off the same way and that we should be able to do the same thing with others to help get them off. Unfortunately, a lot of fake orgasms and lack of attention from partners has resulted in this myth being perpetuated. With this exercise, you're going to create the map of your own pleasure. What "buttons" need to be pushed, how hard, and with what tools?

Use the sexual response cycle map you created in the Sexual Response Cycle chapter: This will help you identify how your body feels when you have orgasms. In this section, I want you to notice what types of sensations you like when you self-pleasure. Do you like a more firm touch or a more gentle touch? What side of your clitoris or penis is more sensitive?

Make a date with yourself: Instead of your self-pleasuring being something you need to "get out of the way," make a date to spend an hour on your self-pleasuring. Try to do this at least once a week. You may find that you reach orgasm quickly and have time left in your hour. You can try to have another orgasm, or you can give yourself a full body massage. Try starting with a full body massage, and work your way toward your genitals, your nipples, your anus, and so forth.

Connect with your partner or a friend: Set a date to talk to either your partner or a close friend about self-pleasuring. Talk about what you like, what you don't like, and experiences you've had. This might feel frightening or difficult at first, but getting into the conversation can be freeing! You might find some new tips or new methods or find something in common.

Goal Check-In: As I mentioned, time can be a big factor when it comes to achieving our goals. Self-pleasuring is an activity that typically requires alone time. If you are finding it difficult to get the homework done, or to find time to spend alone, consider making it a goal to schedule time for yourself. Put it into your calendar so that you know you have set specific time aside for it.

SEVEN ● ● ● ● ● ●

Sex Toys

Sex toys have been around since the late nineteenth century, yet they're still a mystery to many people. I break down the different types of toys available and talk about how to integrate toys into your sexual practice and how to use them for mutual orgasm. Toys can be a huge asset in the bedroom, and with a little bit of additional information, they might be that extra little push needed to take your orgasms from OK to "Oh, wow!"

So you want to have orgasms together during sex, including during penetrative sex. In reality, male and female bodies are not always going to line up perfectly to achieve orgasm through penetration alone. As mentioned in the Anatomy and Physiology chapter (page 32), for many women, their clitoris needs continuous, direct stimulation in order for orgasm to take place. So how can women have orgasms with their partners during penetrative sex? One answer is to use vibrating sex toys.

Sex toys have long been given a bad rap. Many people feel that if they require the use of sex toys, they're doing something wrong or the sex toy will replace the need for partners. This couldn't be further from the truth! Sex toys are a wonderful invention that can help enhance sexual function and pleasure.

Sex toys can be used alone or with a partner. Over the past few years, many new types have come on to the market with the specific purpose of being used for partnered intercourse.

These toys can be used to help partners achieve orgasm simultaneously, though they still require communication between partners.

LUBRICANT

Lubricant is one of the most underused and underrated products available. Using lubricant can make everything feel more sensitive, more slippery, and more connected. Can you see how this is going to be beneficial as you try to have simultaneous orgasms?

Choosing the right lubricant can be a bit of a challenge, but most sex toy stores and even a few pharmacies carry decent lubricants. What you're looking for in a lubricant is one that will retain its lubricating properties and won't dry out quickly. The difficulty is that everyone's body reacts slightly differently with lubricants, and it might take a few tries to find the right lubricant for you and your partner. Thankfully, lubricant companies have figured this out and created "pillow packs," or single-use packages, that you can try out to see what works.

If you find that you've had a lot of irritation using lubricant in the past, look for a lubricant that's glycerin-free. For some women, glycerin can cause discomfort, burning, yeast infections, urinary tract infections, microscopic tears to the vaginal tissue, and rashes. Not all women experience these symptoms, but if they do occur, it's worth getting it checked out by your health care professional. He or she can determine whether the lube is the cause of the discomfort.

If you're looking for a longer-lasting lubricant, consider trying a silicone-based one. The silicone-based lubricant will stay slipperier longer, and most people don't find that the silicone lube irritates them in any way. The downside to silicone lubricants is that they can't be used in direct contact with silicone sex toys, because the silicone lubricant can damage the toy's silicone material. On a side note, a sexologist I went to school with specializes in pelvic pain, including vulvodynia and vaginismus, and her recommendation for women experiencing any type of pelvic pain is to use a silicone-based lubricant like Pujr or Eros.

THE WE-VIBE

The We-Vibe is a new and innovative vibrator that can be worn internally and externally. One side fits on the inside of the woman's vagina, and the other side sits on her clitoris. Because of the way the vibrator is designed, it's small enough that the woman can still have penetrative sex while wearing the vibrator internally. The We-Vibe is designed to hit the G-spot and the clitoris at the same time.

This is a great option for couples interested in having sex with a vibrator because they don't have too much to worry about in terms of positioning, holding, or moving around. The added benefit is that the extra friction and sensation for the male partner might increase his orgasm as well.

It might take a little time to get comfortable using this vibrator, since it's a different sensation to have a vibrator in the vagina at the same time as having penetrative sex. However, the We-Vibe is continuously one of the top-rated vibrators for a reason: it works!

THE HITACHI MAGIC WAND

The tried, tested, and true vibrator! It's been around for a long time, is extremely powerful, and is a favorite of many experts in the sexuality field. The reason that it's popular is that it combines a lot of different factors that people look for in a vibrator. It has two speeds, both of which are quite powerful; it has a large surface area; and several attachments have been

● ● ● ● ● ● ● ● ● ● ● ● ● ● ● ● ●

She says . . .

I have a hard time having orgasms through sex, but not by myself or with a vibrator. If I could use a vibrator when I'm having sex with my partner, I think I could probably have an orgasm, but I'm worried he might think using a vibrator would mean he's not good enough.

Suggestion:

In a nonconfrontational way, sit down with your partner and suggest that you go shopping for a sex toy together. With the new toys these days, there are lots of options, and many of them are less intimidating.

Encouraging your partner to use the sex toy with you will include him further in the use of the vibrator and can help him learn how he can use the vibrator to help you achieve orgasm. After that, you can continue to try new things with the vibrator and build up to using it together to help achieve simultaneous orgasms.

● ● ● ● ● ● ● ● ● ● ● ● ● ● ● ● ●

made to allow it to be not only a clitoral vibrator but also a G-spot stimulator. It's also an electrical toy, which for some people is a huge benefit, but for others it's a significant downside. The fact that it plugs into a wall socket limits where the vibrator can be used, but as a result it also has a more powerful motor and a longer life span than most toys.

The size of the Hitachi Magic Wand makes it more difficult to use in certain positions, such as the missionary position, but the longer handle makes it easier to use in other positions, like the rear-entry position.

Some people find the strong vibrations to be too strong when they're starting out. One solution is to wrap the vibrator in a soft towel to dampen the sensation.

VIBRATING RINGS

In recent years, vibrating penis rings have made their way into the sex toy stores and some pharmacies as well. They're versatile and serve two purposes to be a penis ring (see the section on penis rings) and to be a vibrator, which can have direct contact with the clitoris for added stimulation. Several condom companies such as Trojan, LifeStyles, and Durex have disposable vibrating rings that can be used several times. The Mio Penis Ring by Je Joue is reusable and rechargeable and has multiple vibration settings. It's sure to become a favorite for couples interested in finding that extra clitoral stimulation they desire.

There are several other types of vibrating penis rings available to fit a variety of budgets and needs. It's important when looking for this type of toy to find something that'll be comfortable for both partners. Although these toys may look intimidating at first, they may be a great addition to your sex life. They're definitely gaining more popularity because of the benefits they offer.

Any vibrating sex toy can be used to stimulate the clitoris externally while penetrative sex is happening; the trick is to find a position with enough space for the toy to be in contact with the clitoris and to allow the user to move the toy around. For suggestions for positions, see the Positions for Men and Women chapter (page 114).

DILDOS

By definition a dildo is a sex toy used for penetration. Dildos come in various shapes, sizes, and materials. Dildos can be used for either vaginal or anal penetration, though the dildos used for anal penetration must have a flared base. The benefit of using one is that the dildo can add a feeling of fullness, which some women enjoy as they reach their climax. In terms of anal penetration, for both women and men, the addition of anal stimulation can intensify their orgasms.

When choosing a dildo, bigger is not always better. Some people prefer to have a smaller size dildo that's more maneuverable, while others prefer a larger size for more pressure. Either way, the dildo's size should not be considered in a comparison with the male partner but as an addition to the sexual repertoire.

FURNITURE

There are several sex-specific pieces of furniture created to help people position themselves better sexually. As I discuss in more detail in the Positions for Men and Women chapter (page 114), elevating the female partner's hips can help create more direct pressure for the clitoris. The addition of furniture can also help make positions more comfortable and adaptable for people with differing levels of flexibility and physical ability.

The Love Bumper, a company based in Vancouver, British Columbia, has taken bedroom ergonomics to a new level and designed different sex cushions to enhance the comfort of sex. Some of their products include pockets where vibrators can be positioned to create direct clitoral stimulation.

BUT I DON'T KNOW HOW TO USE A VIBRATOR!

When people make their first foray into using sex toys it can sometimes be daunting, scary, weird, or just plain uncomfortable. How do you use a sex toy? How do you learn how to do it properly?

The first step is to understand what the sex toy is going to feel like on your body. One simple way is to test the vibration against your nose. It might seem silly to hold a sex toy up to your nose to figure it out, but at most reputable sex toy stores, they won't even bat an eye if you try this. This might sound like an excellent way to pass on germs, but most stores have sex toy cleaners and can wipe the surface of the toy before and after you hold it up to your nose. If you find that the vibration is too strong on your nose, you might find it to be too strong on your genitals.

For most beginners, buying a toy with variable speeds might be the way to go. As your body gets to know the vibrations, you might find you need a slightly stronger vibration than you originally thought. Take your time getting to know the different buttons and settings on the vibrator, as this will save you the effort later when you're going for the orgasm.

For women using a vibrator the first time, the temptation might be to go straight for the clitoris and go to town. There's nothing wrong with that, because it feels great. However, another method is to explore the entire body, starting slowly around the neck, breasts, nipples, and working your way down to the genitals. Take your time, and explore all of the erogenous zones.

Try different positions: lying on your back, lying on your front, squatting, legs up, legs down, legs together, legs apart. You might find that the vibrator provides different sensations for each position.

If you find that the vibrator is too intense, you can use a soft cloth or towel or a nice soft fabric between your skin and the vibrator. Some people find that having jeans on actually intensifies the feeling, as the vibration spreads over a wider area of the genitals.

PURCHASING A SEX TOY TO USE WITH YOUR PARTNER

I remember watching the original *American Pie* movie. In one scene a character is reading *The Ultimate Sex Bible,* and one page features a vibrator and the words "know thy enemy" are written below it. I don't know exactly how the rumors started that sex toys are the enemy, but they're most definitely not the enemy. If anything, vibrators should be seen as members of the team! Sure, there are some situations where someone might become more reliant on the vibrator for pleasure than they are on their partner, but most people enjoy the human connection that they have with their partner more than the time they spend with the battery-operated vibrator they might enjoy every once in a while.

More often than not, it's about finding the right sex toy to use with a partner. But the toy people use together might not be the same toy that they use by themselves. It is OK to have more than one sex toy. Many people have several toys that serve different purposes.

The vibrator selection out there is vast, and it's easy to get lost with all of the beautiful colors and funky shapes available. Function is always the primary goal. When looking for a toy to use with a partner, you should keep in mind these keys.

What position do you generally like to have sex in?

If you're most comfortable having sex in the missionary position, a Hitachi Magic Wand may not be the best choice for a partnered sex toy. If you like positions that require your bodies to be close together, you may be better off choosing a toy that can be worn on the penis, like the Mio Penis ring by Je Joue, or an internal and external vibrator, like the We-Vibe.

Are you looking for an internal or external vibrator?

In general, vibrators can be used internally or externally, and some of them are dual purpose. Some people like having the ability to have both purposes met in one toy while other people prefer to have different vibrators. There are also the dual-headed vibrators like the Rabbit that have internal and clitoral stimulators. The consideration here needs to be what you'll be using the toy for. Look for a toy that's easily maneuverable and comfortable to hold, with accessible controls.

Do you want the toy to be dual in purpose?

If both partners are interested in using the toy for pleasure, bringing your partner to the sex toy store or browsing the selection online together is a good idea. Not all vibrators are built with male pleasure in mind, but there are some toys that work for both men and women, and can be used together to provide additional pleasure for both partners.

What types of materials are you looking for?

Not all vibrators are created equal. In recent years, sex toys have gone high-tech, with a focus on pleasure and an increased awareness of the types of materials used.

Unfortunately, there are still sex toys available made with materials that are not good for the body, especially the genital tissue, which is more delicate than other types of skin. These toys are often marketed as novelty toys and are made with a chemical called phthalate. Instead of these "jelly" toys, look for toys made of silicone, hard plastic, ceramic, Lucite, acrylic, or metal, or another Food and Drug Administration–approved material, such as CyberSkin, the material used in the FleshLight.

Phthalates

Avoid these toys at all costs! Phthalates are unsafe for the body and, when used on the vulva or in the vagina, can leak toxins into the body. It's true that they're generally less expensive, but spending a bit more on a toy that will last longer and be safer on your genitals is an investment worth making!

Stores like Womyn's Ware in Vancouver, Come as You Are and Good for Her in Toronto, Good Vibrations in San Francisco and Boston, and Babeland Toys in Seattle offer a great selection of phthalate-free toy options, and they have shipping options. Most reputable sex toy stores do not sell toys with phthalates. If you do have questions, ask the store employees, and if you don't get a satisfactory answer, move on!

A WORD ABOUT PENIS RINGS

A penis ring, also called a cock ring, can be an incredibly versatile product that couples can use together. There are a few benefits to using a cock ring, but also a few precautions to be aware of. Penis rings can be made of various materials, but the safest type is generally a stretchy silicone rubber. For most beginners, metal is not a preferred option, as the metal has no give and can be difficult to remove. Additionally, it's better to purchase penis rings from sex toy stores rather than to use materials that look as if they might work; more than one person has ended up in the emergency room as a result of using different materials that seem like a good cheap solution. Trust me when I say metal piping does not make a good penis ring!

Penis rings can help men maintain erections longer because it slows the flow of blood from the erectile tissue. This can be a great benefit in delaying the orgasm to time it better with a partner. It can also help men maintain a firmer erection for a longer period of time.

When using a penis ring, men should be aware that they need to be careful about putting it on, and about how long they wear it. Start by leaving the ring on for five minutes, and build up to a maximum of thirty minutes. If at any time the user begins to feel numbness or sensations like pins and needles in his penis, he should immediately remove the ring.

The penis ring can be placed around the shaft of the penis at the base or around the shaft and testicles, depending on the user's comfort.

If someone is using a penis ring made out of a more rigid material, it's better to put the testicles through the ring first and then put the flaccid penis through the ring. When the ring is made out of a rigid material like metal, it's not a good idea to put the ring on when the penis is erect. If the ring is made out of a softer and stretchier material like silicone, the user can choose to put it on either when he's flaccid or when he's erect.

There are many variations of cock rings, and they come in a range of different costs The most basic models can be purchased for about five dollars. There are cock rings available with vibrators, which can act as clitoral stimulators and aid in helping the female partner reach orgasm.

USING SEX TOYS TOGETHER

As I mentioned already, seeing sex toys as something detrimental to your sex life isn't going to help anyone, especially if you're trying to achieve simultaneous orgasms. Sex toys can be the best tool in your sexual tool kit for reaching orgasms, whether it's alone, with a partner, or with penetrative sex.

When using a toy, everyone has a different approach. The toy might feel different depending on how it's used, and this is something to be aware of when using it for simultaneous orgasm timing. If you're using it alone, you might be positioning your body in a way that's hitting different parts of the toy on different parts of your body. If you're using it with a partner, you might need to hold it differently or be positioned differently.

Try having the female partner control it on her body, then have her partner use the toy on her body. Next, try using the vibrator together while stimulating the other partner manually. This will give you a better idea of how you'll experience the pleasure, but also how you'll give pleasure while receiving pleasure. The next step is to use the vibrator during penetra-

91

She says . . .

My partner and I are able to have orgasms, but a lot of the time he'll have an orgasm first, and afterward I'll have to use a vibrator to have my own orgasm. It doesn't bother me, but it would be really nice if we could have our climax together.

He says . . .

Sometimes my orgasm sneaks up on me, and I'm not ready to have one, but it happens anyway. When that happens, I know she hasn't had her orgasm yet, and although I know she's not angry with me, I know she'd like it if we could climax together.

Suggestion:

Using a sex toy during penetrative sex can help this couple achieve orgasms together. It's also worth remembering that women have a much shorter refractory period than men, and if she has one orgasm, she might be able to have another one timed with his.

If he does have his orgasm first, they might want to try using the vibrator together for her to have her orgasm, so that they're both involved in the process. This can help them for next time by adding to their building verbal and nonverbal communication cues about their orgasms together.

tive sex. Again, depending on the toy, you might find that you need to position yourself differently to feel the sensation from the vibrator and to be able to reach the right spots. The female partner might find that as she gets closer to orgasm, she wants to keep the vibrator on her clitoris, or she might want to move the vibrator and have her partner's body stimulate her to orgasm.

Be aware that as the vibrator is on her genitals, the male partner may also notice some additional vibrations, and this can intensify his sensation and might change his orgasm cycle and sexual response. Obviously this might result in the need to reevaluate timing, and that's OK! Eventually, using this method might be your method of choice, as it can help the female partner reach orgasm more easily with the vibrator.

SUMMARY

Sex toys can be useful in so many ways when it comes to sex and, especially, in helping couples sync their orgasms. Because women typically need direct clitoral stimulation to achieve clitoral orgasms, sex toys can make this happen more easily. For women who need more time than they usually have through penetrative sex alone, using a vibrator can help them achieve orgasms more quickly. Using a vibrator may take some time to get used to, but once couples are comfortable with integrating the orgasm into their sex lives, they may find that it gives them the extra boost needed to have simultaneous orgasms!

Simultaneous O

⬤ HOMEWORK ⬤

Toys R Us: For this homework assignment, you'll need to either venture out to a reputable sex toy store for your toy or purchase one online (for a complete list, check the reference section at the end of the book). I've given you the outline of some of the different toys, but because everyone's body is different, you might need to experiment a bit to find one that matches your needs. Your homework assignment is to find a sex toy that suits your needs and that you and your partner can use together.

Got the toy, now what? The next step is to identify what type of stimulation you like. Both women and men might enjoy stimulation, vibration, pressure, and so forth, but again, since everyone's body is different, you might find you need a different type of pressure or stimulation from the toy to reach orgasm.

Try it together! Try using the toy with your partner. Your partner can watch you use the toy or can try holding the toy to bring you to orgasm. Enjoy this part of the process; it's meant to be fun and pleasurable for you.

Goal Check-In: It can be very intimidating to buy a toy, and to use it! If you've never considered using a toy, but are interested in learning more, make a goal for yourself to not only purchase the toy, but to use it to stimulate yourself or your partner to orgasm.

EIGHT   ●   ●   ●   ●   ●   ●

Oral Sex

There's so much to be said about oral sex, yet there's still so much that people aren't willing to talk about! Well, here's the deal. When it comes to simultaneous orgasms, oral sex may be the easiest way to get there. Oral sex offers the opportunity to pace what you're doing, add more or less pressure, and to work together with your partner to determine how it feels for him or her and for you!

The issue is, how do we do it properly? One of the best aspects of oral sex is that using the mouth is often more specific and, for some, more pleasant than the touch of fingers. Also, moving bodies into different positions to use mouths, hands, and genitals is fun to do. The difficult part is knowing what needs to be done. I'll identify the different methods and how to do both one-on-one oral sex and mutual oral sex.

Let's start with the basics and build from there.

ORAL SEX ON
A MALE PARTNER

For many men, receiving oral sex is at the top of their favorite sexual activities. It's extremely pleasurable and it offers a different sensation than manual or penetrative sex.

Communication is key: To make oral sex more pleasurable for your partner, ask him what he does and doesn't enjoy. The truth is, every penis likes something slightly different. You might be great at giving a blow job to one guy, but another guy might not love your technique as much. Find the pleasure for your guy by asking for tips. If you approach it this way, you won't be disappointed or hurt when he makes suggestions.

Use your tongue: Using your tongue can increase sensation and make it feel as if you're doing a lot more with just a little more effort.

Give yourself a break! A lot of women say that they hate giving blow jobs because their jaws start to hurt after a while. Take time to build up your oral skills. Relax your jaw as much as you can, and don't feel as if you have to be a deep-throating expert immediately. You can take breaks, and take your time to gain more endurance.

Use your hand: By using your hand, you can add to the sensation and also make him feel as if you're getting deeper than you are. Also, using your hand to stroke and grab his testicles can add to his pleasure; just make sure you check with him first to make sure he likes it!

Play with his testicles, his perineum, and his anus: Using your free hand to touch his erogenous zones can help him break through a plateau and increase pleasure substantially. Some men love the surprise of being touched in new places or with new strokes, but other men might find it uncomfortable or even violating to be touched in these places. Make sure you use your pleasure checklist beforehand to find out if these types of touches are OK or out of bounds.

Think of his penis like an ice cream cone or Popsicle: Lick with your tongue before taking his whole penis into your mouth. This will prime him, excite him, and prepare him for the sensations. Changing back and forth between lick-ing and sucking is a great way to tease him, and changing the sensations will bring him to the brink and back several times.

If you find something that works, keep going: If your man is sending you signals to indicate that what you're doing is working, keep going. If you want to experiment with timing and see how far you can push him to the brink of orgasm and back, this is the time to do it! Afterward, he can tell you how the sensation felt for him and identify which sensations were the ones that pushed him closer to climax.

Don't be afraid to try something new: Try a different position, such as from the side, standing, kneeling, "69," or another position that you might think is going to give you a better angle. Men like having a different view of your body, and changing it up might give him the visual pleasure he craves. Watching your mouth engulf his penis is quite often a highlight of receiving oral sex.

Be aware of his cues: Each man has different O faces and movements. If he starts throwing his head back with his eyes closed, grabbing your hair, thrusting his hips, or moving in a different way, he might be closer to orgasm. For some guys, in this stage it's hard to communicate how close they are. If this is the first time you're giving him a blow job, consider continuing to do what you're doing to see what happens. Afterward, you can discuss the possibility that when he gets to that stage, you can pull back a bit and see if he can control his orgasm.

Spitting or swallowing: Everyone has a different opinion on whether to spit or swallow, and everyone is entitled to their own opinion. Each option is OK and won't cause harm physically. If someone has a sensitive gag reflex, swallowing might not feel great. If someone has sensitive tastes, swallowing also might not be the preferred option. Some people enjoy swallowing their partner's ejaculate, because for them this is part of the experience and highly erotic. Whatever you decide, make sure you're both comfortable with it. And if you

Simultaneous O

decide not to swallow, don't make a big production of spitting the ejaculate out; it can be done discreetly, without making it into a negative experience, which is the last thing someone would want after a mind-blowing orgasm!

ORAL SEX ON A FEMALE PARTNER

One of the great mysteries is why oral sex on a woman is so seldom discussed. I remember being quite young and having a good idea of what a blow job was, but "going down" on a woman was something I didn't quite grasp. For many women, until it happens to them, they don't understand how amazing it can feel. Some women have fears about how their genitals smell or taste, and so they can't relax and enjoy oral sex. Please note: The pH of a woman's vulva is acidic, and most women will have a taste that's similar to plain yogurt or a dry chardonnay. It's different from any other taste in the world, and that's OK, but it might take some time to get used to or to enjoy.

This should never be something that we make into a negative. I would imagine that most people don't love wine the first time they taste it, and a woman's body is probably not much different. There are flavored lubricants that can mask the taste, but most of them contain sugar, which is not good for the vulva, so I recommend skipping them if at all possible.

Instead of making it a negative, I'd like to see this become a positive, and have women be free to enjoy the pleasures of oral sex. Here are some tips to make oral sex more enjoyable for your partner.

Find a position that's comfortable for both of you: One of the most common complaints I've heard about oral sex is that it's uncomfortable. Try using pillows to prop up your partner's hips to make her vulva more accessible.

98

Use big strokes to start with: You want to use the whole surface of your tongue to stroke the maximum surface on her vulva. Incorporate the labia and the clitoris, but don't put too much pressure on the clitoris at first. For many women, this can be much too sensitive to start with and might even be uncomfortable until they're fully aroused.

Use your fingers as necessary: Having pressure in her vagina can help a woman get closer to orgasm. The feeling of pressure and fullness helps increase sensation. Some women like their partner to move their fingers in and out of their vagina, while others just want the pressure of fullness with no movement. If this is uncomfortable for you to do, consider using a dildo or vibrator to create that pressure.

The case of the disappearing clitoris: For some women, as they get closer to orgasm, the engorgement and erectile tissue will actually lift the clitoris and pull it into the body. This is often mistaken as a sign that the woman is losing arousal. This is not the case! Instead, keep doing what you're doing! This is a sign that what you're doing is working!

Pointed tongue: As your partner gets closer to orgasm, you might want to change your technique and use a more pointed tongue to directly stimulate the clitoris. This can increase pleasure and help your partner to get over the plateau to orgasm.

Communication: Similar to men, women might get to a point where they're unable to communicate how they're feeling. They might be using physical cues instead of verbal cues to indicate that things are feeling amazing. If this starts happening, go with what you're doing and later discuss what did and didn't work for her.

Don't stop: No, seriously, when you get to the point where what you're doing is working, if you change it up, you might throw her out of her sexual response cycle and lose all progress. It might seem tempting to try something different, but the clitoris is a finicky organ, and by changing up your technique at that critical moment, you might have to start all over.

NEVER EVER EVER: Do not, under any circumstances, blow air into your partner's vagina. This can cause an embolism, and can even cause death. Not exactly what you're looking for during oral sex.

Keep a towel by the bed: When you add saliva to vaginal lubrication, you could end up with quite a lot of liquid. For some people, this amount of liquid actually takes away from the experience. You might find that a quick wipe helps bring more sensation to your partner. Just make sure you check in with her first that this is OK, as it might feel like an insult if done without permission.

Explore other areas: Try using your free hand to explore her perineum, anus, breasts, inner thighs, stomach, and so forth. By touching these erogenous zones, you might help get her over the plateau and into orgasm. But, as I said above with oral sex on a man, make sure you have permission to do this type of exploring, so that it feels comfortable and not violating.

EXPLORING ORAL SEX TOGETHER

Oral sex can be so rewarding when done properly. It can be an appetizer or a main course! By communicating your wants and needs, oral sex can be used to reach simultaneous orgasm with your partner.

Using the "69" Position

Although this is the most common position, it can be challenging at first. Positioning yourself so that both you and your

She says . . .

After incorporating other options into our sex lives, both of us are a lot happier. We started out by exploring mutual oral sex, and we were able to use that to start both having orgasms. By communicating afterward, we were able to see when the other was getting close and how to change up our timing to accommodate that. At first it was difficult; when we started doing this, we got lost in our own pleasure or started worrying that we weren't doing enough and weren't able to enjoy ourselves. With some practice, we got it right!

Suggestion:

Having simultaneous oral sex can be a wonderful feeling. As she says, at first it can be a challenge to relax into the sensations, but practicing and having fun together can help move past this challenge. Being aware of how the other person is feeling can both enhance and distract from your own sensations, but for some people, when they notice their partner getting closer, they find themselves being pulled along into the next phase of the sexual response cycle!

partner are comfortable enough to experience pleasure can be tricky. Some people find that using pillows to prop themselves up can make them significantly more comfortable.

Having one person on top and one person on the bottom can work well. For most couples, the easiest option in this position is to have the female partner on top. This allows her to control the depth she uses for oral sex on her male partner. She can also lower herself into position so that her partner doesn't have to raise his head up too much to perform oral sex on her. There are many variations to this position, and using pillows and chairs to prop hips up can be more comfortable for people and help them to maintain this position for longer times.

Another option is to have both partners lying on their sides. This can work quite well, but you might require some pillows to help prop your heads up; another option is to have your head resting on your partner's leg. When people are concentrating on holding their heads up, it can distract from the pleasure they're experiencing.

Some couples are eager to try out more adventurous positions, where they're holding each other upside down. For very few people, the extremeness of this position might be stimulating, but for most people, trying to hold this position is going to be unrealistic and uncomfortable. The goal of enjoying oral sex is not to end up with a muscle cramp or back pain! Find a position you like, and if you find yourself straining to hold the position, use some pillows or props to help you sustain the position with comfort. The last thing you want is for the position to distract you from pleasure.

Build Up to Mutual Oral Sex

Oral sex can also be enjoyed with one person performing oral sex at a time, building up to orgasm. For many people, performing oral sex on their partner is a significant stimulation and gets them pretty close to the plateau phase without any stimulation. It's very hot to watch your partner enjoy receiving the pleasure that you're providing. As you build up to orgasm, you can move into the "69" position and stimulate each other to orgasm.

This method makes it easy to sync your orgasms, because the person who's receiving oral sex can verbalize how close he or she is or can use hand signals to encourage his or her partner to move into the "69" position.

Oral sex and manual stimulation—a match made in heaven!

When people find mutual oral sex to be too intense, or the position to be uncomfortable, another option is to pair oral sex with manual stimulation.

One option is to have the male partner lie down on his back. The woman straddles his head, facing his lower body. In this position, she can kneel over his head while stimulating his penis with her hands. As she feels herself closing in on her climax, she can speed up her strokes on his penis with her hands and bring him to his orgasm as she reaches hers.

Another option is to have the male partner lie on his back. His partner can lie down perpendicular to his body. In this position, his partner has full access to perform oral sex while he stimulates her genitals with his hand.

COMBINING ORAL SEX AND SEX TOYS

One of the major bonuses of sex toys is that they allow for a connection without much work. When people have difficulty focusing on having orgasms and stimulating their partner to orgasm at the same time, using a sex toy can help solve this issue. Using a sex toy with a longer handle that's easy to maneuver can keep the connection between partners, but needs less focus, freeing both partners to enjoy pleasure.

Sex toys can be used in any of the above positions to help couples achieve orgasms together.

One thing to note is that there are some really excellent books out there dedicated specifically to oral sex. If you want a more detailed account or are looking for more information on this particular sex skill, check out the reference section.

SUMMARY

Oral sex can be an excellent tool for couples looking to achieve simultaneous orgasms. Much like with manual sex (using your hands to stimulate your partner), couples can have more control over the contact they have with their partner's genitals. The mouth and tongue are almost as deft as the fingers and hands and provide a unique sensation.

Many people enjoy oral sex more than penetrative sex. The sensations can vary through the type of movements, and using the tongue can change the sensation further.

One or both partners can enjoy oral sex together, and this adds an excellent benefit for people trying to achieve simultaneous orgasm.

☛ HOMEWORK ☚

Oral Sex Sexual Response: Using the sexual response cycle, see how your orgasms vary from self-pleasuring when you're having oral sex.

Make it your main meal: Instead of using oral sex as a warm-up or as foreplay, experiment with making it your main course with your partner once a week. Oral sex, like other types of sex, will become easier as you practice more. When you get more experienced with it, you might notice that it becomes very pleasurable to give and receive oral sex.

Goal Check-In: Oral sex skills might be something that you or your partner is interested in acquiring or improving on. Because many people find oral sex so pleasurable, you might want to make a goal of having an oral sex–only session or sessions.

Considerations for Penetrative Sex

Sadly, one of the biggest myths about sex is that partnered sex between men and women should always yield orgasm through hard and fast penetration. We have multiple sources to thank for this, starting with Sigmund Freud and continuing with our current media environment and the availability of pornographic material. Missionary position may result in simultaneous orgasms for some people, but ultimately for most people, other things need to be in play for this to happen. In this chapter, we'll go over some external factors that can help people achieve simultaneous orgasms and what it takes to get there.

We'll also look at some warm-up ideas before penetrative sex and identify warm-up penetrative positions to help both partners get ready to time their orgasms.

When it comes to positions, anything that can be imagined can be tried, but they're not all necessarily comfortable or a precursor to simultaneous orgasm. One major factor people seem to forget when they create "the position of the week" or browse a book of outrageous positions is that they might actually not be comfortable for everyone to perform. So you have to try them out. Let your body and your partner's body be the guide to which positions are best for you. Just because a magazine or book recommends a position doesn't mean that it'll be great for everyone.

THE VISUAL FACTOR

When we're thinking of penetrative sex, one big consideration needs to be the visual factor. What visual stimulation are you receiving? Are you able to see your partner's face? Is what you're looking at affecting the sexual response?

For some couples, looking into each other's eyes is a necessity when they're having sex because it helps to connect them. It acts almost as a grounding factor as well as an intense connection. Other couples don't need this type of connection and can instead use blindfolds, positions where they're facing away from each other, and so forth.

The other part of the visual factor is what each person is looking at during sex. As I mentioned in the Oral Sex chapter (page 95), it can be incredibly hot to be able to see the other person and what he or she is doing. For example, some people love watching the thrusts as the penis enters the vagina, and the sensation that goes with that can be unbelievable as they watch and feel it. In the rear-entry position, the female partner may be relaxed and able to have an orgasm because she knows her partner isn't looking at her face, or she might have a more difficult time reaching orgasm because she can't see her partner and is looking at the wall or at a pillow. Be aware of how the visual stimulation can alter the sensations.

THE KISSING FACTOR

Another matter of preference for some couples is being able to kiss while having penetrative sex; for others, being prevented from kissing elevates the passion, intensity, and primal nature of sex. Kissing is an intimate activity, and depending on the mood of the partners, it may create a deeper connection that allows them to orgasm together. Or not kissing may allow them to be more animalistic with more intense penetration, which can bring them to orgasm together.

PENETRATIVE SEX POSITIONS

Have you ever flipped through the magazines at the grocery store checkout only to wonder, "How is it possible that *Cosmo* comes up with a new position every month?" It's remarkable, really, that there are so many positions and so much variety to the positions. Unfortunately, for most couples, the variety in these positions isn't necessarily going to be possible, and very few of them will lead to simultaneous orgasm.

He says...

My girlfriend reads a lot of magazines that have information about sex and sexual positions. Sometimes I feel like the suggested positions in these magazines aren't possible, and if they are, they don't feel good, or we spend so much time and energy trying to get into them that we don't end up enjoying sex. Is there anything wrong with just having sex in positions we're comfortable with?

Suggestion:

There is nothing wrong with having sex in positions that you are comfortable with, as long as both of you are enjoying those positions. It's nice for couples to have a position that they can use as their "go-to" or starting position. Trying other positions can add some excitement and can also give you both the opportunity to find what works best for simultaneous orgasms.

If you're finding that you're trying positions that require you to be a contortionist, or to hold your partner up for long periods of time, those positions might not be as much for pleasure as they are for a challenge. Check in with your partner to find out what positions she likes for sexual pleasure and which she likes for excitement. Don't be afraid to ditch the suggestions the magazines make and instead focus on what it is that works for you and your partner.

In the next chapter, I recommend some positions that will work for people, but be aware that not every position works for everyone, and you might have to improvise, try different positions, and change things up every once in a while.

For more on how to sync orgasms, the next chapter touches on positions that will encourage orgasms and delay orgasms. While these positions will help you and your partner to start your simultaneous orgasm journey through penetrative sex, it's up to you and your partner to be aware of how the positions work for you.

Because everyone's bodies are different, we also have different areas that are more sensitive and those that are less sensitive. Using the keys in the previous chapters to identify your own sexual response cycle in combination with these positions will help you reach your goals. It's best to think of these sections as a jumping-off point, and if you need more variety to your positions—before you run out to buy an gigantic book of positions—use your own imagination, work with your partner, and create what it is that you need for yourselves.

For most men, orgasms happen when there's adequate stimulation and friction to the penis. The head and frenulum tend to be the most sensitive part of the shaft. So positions that provide less friction and stimulation are going to be positions that delay orgasms.

As men age, they tend to have more of a delay in orgasm and in some cases find it difficult to orgasm. Some men also might find it difficult to have an erection. If these are issues you or your partner is experiencing, read the Troubleshooting chapter (page 128).

WARM-UP FOR PENETRATIVE SEX

When warming up for penetrative sex, you might find that you and your partner are already at varied stages of your sexual response cycles. This is common, but it can cause one partner to reach climax before the other one has even hit the plateau.

The first consideration is whether you want to use other types of sex for warm-up. Manual sex, mutual masturbation, oral sex, and anal stimulation can all be used as warm-up positions to penetrative sex. Couples can use these methods to sync their sexual response cycles.

Another position that couples can use is a really good make-out. Intertwining your bodies, touching different parts of the body, sharing deep passionate kisses, and teasing each other with no genital stimulation can heighten the erotic sensations and build tension before penetration starts.

Using manual sex can be a great warm-up for penetrative sex. Using your hands to stimulate your partner can be very beneficial and can help gauge how far you can get into the sexual response cycle with manual sex. This connects to the idea I mentioned in the Self-Pleasuring chapter (page 72): most people know their own bodies best through masturbation, and using the hands can help trigger the awareness of their own sexual response cycle.

The next warm-up position is often referred to as dry sex, but it can be highly pleasurable despite its name. Grinding the hips together without penetration can result in lots of direct clitoral contact, as well as a less intense stimulation to the penis. Because this position can give adequate sensation to the clitoris, it can also bring the woman further into her sexual response while keeping the man's sexual response under control.

PENETRATIVE POSITIONS FOR WARM-UP

If you're looking to have a longer sexual experience, warming up with penetrative sex can be used to help the female partner warm up comfortably and raise her sexual response through penetration. But the penetrative position also needs to be a position where the male partner is not overly stimulated and too quickly aroused. To have penetrative sex, men need to have a firm enough erection to penetrate their partner. In some cases, this means that they might already be two steps ahead in the sexual response cycle than their female partner. This is something that needs to be considered in order to sync the sexual response cycles properly.

To start penetrative sex with the intent of simultaneous orgasm, it's best to find a comfortable position that can be easily maintained, with not too much stimulation for either person. Many people consider missionary position a great starting place: it's connected yet doesn't result in a lot of visual stimulation. By having a position that's comfortable to start in, people can get their rhythm together, without raising their sexual arousal to the point where they will mis-time their sexual response cycles.

Finding a position that can be maintained yet also easily changed to different positions will take time, but remembering that for many people that first thrust can be very exciting and sensitized can help them remember to go slow and be aware of the speed and depth of penetration.

LUBRICANT DURING PENETRATIVE SEX

As I discussed in the Sexual Response Cycle chapter (page 57), we need to remember that people can jump in and out of the SRC at different stages. Sometimes women have difficulty producing an adequate amount of lubrication themselves, so to have comfortable penetrative sex, they might need to use additional lubricant.

The use of lubricant might also help her with jump-starting her sexual response cycle, especially with penetrative sex. If you don't have a lot of time to have sex, consider using a lubricant to add to her pleasure and aid in ease of penetration. Using a lubricant can also help reduce friction, which is beneficial to both partners to help identify sensations and to allow for timing orgasms.

SUMMARY

When having penetrative sex with a partner, many different factors aside from penetration itself can affect how people experience pleasure and orgasm. When people initially start having sex at the beginning of a relationship, the external factors are often minimized by excitement and passion. But as the relationship develops over time, external factors become much more important to the pleasure of both partners. It is important to be aware of the factors that will provide a mutually pleasurable experience for you and your partner. Utilizing warm-up positions, kissing, touching, and lubricant can result in more connection and better sexual communication, which can lead to simultaneous orgasms.

⬤ HOMEWORK ⬤

Identifying your sexual pattern: Every couple has a slightly different way of doing things sexually. Some people enjoy a long massage before sex, others enjoy lots of kissing during sex. What is it that you and your partner like to do when you have sex that makes it yours? It doesn't have to be the same every time, but try to identify the signatures of your sexual relationship.

Identify your go-to warm-up position: What position do you and your partner enjoy starting in? Do you start with penetrative sex, or do you start with manual or oral stimulation? Work together to find out what the best options for both of you will be as you move toward simultaneous orgasm.

Set a make-out date: Make a date with your partner to have a really good make-out. Penetration isn't the only way for couples to enjoy themselves, and by having a great make-out session, partners can find the non-genital-focused ways to turn their partner on. Use your hands, your mouth, and your bodies to excite each other.

Goal Check-In: This chapter offers a lot of information that can be useful in working toward your long-term goals. Being aware of these factors can have a positive impact on the relationship you have with your partner as well as the sexual pleasure you both experience. Consider incorporating some of these concepts into the steps you take toward your short-term goals.

TEN ● ● ● ● ● ● ●

Positions for Men and Women

In this chapter, first we'll talk about positions that can help men delay orgasms so that they can sync with their female partners, and we'll also look at positions that can increase men's sexual response to encourage orgasms. Then we'll look into positions that might help women increase their sexual response and desire, in order to prepare their bodies as they build toward plateau without tipping completely over the edge before they're ready. Then we'll discuss positions that women can use to help encourage orgasms.

POSITIONS FOR ENCOURAGING ORGASM IN MEN

As a general rule, the faster the thrusts, and the more friction, the more easily a man will achieve his climax. When a man is looking to climax, almost any position will be sufficient, with those factors in mind. Of course, when he has a partner to be aware of too, it can become a bit more difficult to find positions that will bring both of them to orgasm together.

Additionally, some men find that being teased, and getting close to orgasm before even beginning penetration can increase the likelihood of them going over the top with their climax very quickly! This can be beneficial if the goal is to have them quickly reach orgasm, but also counterproductive if they're trying to last longer with penetrative sex.

Positions for Man on Top

When the man is on top, he can control the speed and depth of his thrusts and can be more in control of the timing of his orgasm.

Missionary position and variations

With the woman lying on her back on the bed, the male partner can lie on top and penetrate from this position. This is one of the most common positions used. There are many variations of this position that can affect the sensation and friction to the penis.

Man on top with legs on outside

In this variation, the male partner has his legs around the woman's legs, and her legs are tightly closed to provide more stimulation to the penis.

The crab

In this variation, the woman is on the bottom, wrapping her legs around the man as he thrusts into her. This can give him deeper penetration and less friction.

Legs up!

Some partners can comfortably have sex in this variation of the missionary position. With the woman on the bottom, she lifts her legs up to her partner's shoulders so he can rest his torso against her legs and get a deeper penetration with more friction.

Positions for the Visual O

Having the ability to see what's happening, watching his penis penetrate his partner, and looking at his partner's body as he's sliding in and out can be an immense turn-on for a man. Having the visual connection to the physical sensation combines the mental and physical in a way that's sure to bring on his orgasm.

Side of the bed

The woman can lie on the bed while the male partner stands at the edge of the bed. Her legs can be elevated, with her heels resting on his shoulders. Using this position allows a full visual for the male partner, as he can see the woman's face, breasts, and genitals, as well as watch his penis enter his partner.

In front of a mirror

Using a mirror to enhance the viewing pleasure of both partners can be a fun addition to many positions. Some men enjoy being able to see their partner's full body in the mirror, which can be achieved by penetration from behind.

On his knees with her wrapped around him

This position has a similar set-up to the side of the bed position. The female partner lies down on the bed. The male partner kneels at her hips, and she can wrap her legs around his hips. As he penetrates, he might find it easiest to gain stability by sliding her up his legs and holding on to her hips or by propping her up with a pillow underneath her back and bottom.

Woman on top

Having the woman in the dominant position where she's able to move the way she needs to can often provide an excellent visual as well as take the control away from the male partner. As the woman moves and thrusts her hips, her partner can give in to the pleasure and experience an intense orgasm.

This position also tends to stimulate the head of the penis and can lead to sudden and intense orgasms.

DELAYING ORGASMS IN MEN

I can't tell you how many times I've heard the adage "think about baseball!" to delay orgasms. If this were possible, men would be able to hold off on orgasms for hours, if not days! Unfortunately, for most men, the only thing this does is take them out of the experience, and their bodies respond to the stimulation rather than to the distracted thoughts.

The best way for a man to delay his orgasm is to be aware of the sensation he's feeling and get well acquainted with the feelings that accompany his sexual response. Many men find that giving the sensations a 1–10 rating is helpful; 1 means not close to orgasm at all, and a 10 is the point of orgasm. Let's face it, for most people sex is an amazing feeling, and it doesn't usually drop much lower than a 5 when penetrative sex is happening. When a man gets to an 8 or 9, it can often be difficult to come back down to a 5, 6, or 7, as he might have passed the point of no return. In that situation, his body takes over and he's unable to stop the cycle to orgasm. As a man approaches the 8 or 9 sensation, it's advisable to change the speed, change the position to help bring the sensation back down to a 6 or 7, or withdraw completely from his partner to bring himself down to a lower level. When this happens, he can continue to manually stimulate his partner so that she doesn't lose her building arousal.

In trying to figure out the sensations and level of approaching orgasm, it's OK to make mistakes. Sometimes, a 9 might feel more like a 6, and then whoops! Orgasm sneaks up really quickly. It might also take some time to get the hang of the sensations and identify them. The best part though? This just means you need to practice more! (Most of my clients don't complain when I tell them they have to have more sex to help them figure out their orgasm cycles!)

Another method that many men have had great success with is to have a "get it out of the way" orgasm. Having the first orgasm allows him to be more relaxed and slightly desensitized. The second orgasm often takes longer and is more controlled when the man is aware of the sensations happening.

The "squeeze technique" is a method that requires men to stop midpenetration and squeeze the head of their penis as they feel themselves getting to the point of orgasm. Although this method is effective, many men don't like it because they have to stop what they're doing, and they're enjoying what they're doing! The additional downside is that this method also requires a pause in whatever sensations the other partner might be enjoying. If that person is moving toward orgasm, a pause might mean he or she is also decreasing how close the orgasm is. This issue can be somewhat mitigated by using a vibrator to help him or her keep the sexual response cycle on track.

Positions That Delay Orgasm in Men

Any position where the man can control the depth and speed of his thrusts will give him additional control.

Missionary position and variations

Although this can also encourage orgasms, having the ability to slow down penetration can also be beneficial.

From behind

Some men find that they can last longer if they can't see their partner's face or be close to them, as it's less of an emotional connection. Their partner can also widen their legs and hips to allow for less friction with the penetration. This position also allows for the female partner to have her clitoris stimulated with ease, and for women who experience G-spot orgasms, this is one of the go-to positions.

When entering his partner from behind, a man is again able to have more control over the depth of his entry and tempo. This position can also lead to a quick orgasm if he's not aware, and if he gives in to the urge to thrust his hips quickly. The female partner is also able to widen her hips to provide less friction.

For some men, this position offers mental stimulation, as it's a position of dominance, and it seems very primal and animalistic. If this happens, this might be a position that needs to be modified.

An additional benefit of this position is that it frees the male partner's hands to provide manual stimulation to his partner's clitoris.

A WORD ABOUT PENISES

When we look at how most men's penises are positioned when erect, the majority point somewhere between the angles of 30 and 120 degrees, with only 5 percent pointing straight up (0 to 30 degrees) and 5 percent pointing straight down (120 to 180 degrees).

When looking at some different sexual positions, it's important to consider what your penis angle is. If the angle is more upward, positions that bend your penis down might feel uncomfortable or strained. If the angle is more downward, you might feel uncomfortable or strained when you try positions that push your penis up.

Try to find positions that look comfortable, and go easy on yourself! Don't try to force yourself into positions. It's a surefire way to either hurt yourself or prevent orgasm from happening.

DELAYING ORGASMS IN WOMEN

Positions for women are a bit trickier to categorize. Women's bodies are all so very different that it's important for each woman to figure out which positions work best for her. The vast majority of women do need additional forms of stimulation during penetration to achieve orgasm. This is not a problem or a reason to feel bad; this is just anatomy, and considerations need to be made. The past few chapters have discussed alternative methods to achieving simultaneous orgasm; using some of those skills will be useful when it comes to encouraging women to achieve orgasm through penetration.

She says...

I've had several different male partners, and I've found that sometimes the angle of his penis has an effect on whether or not I can have an orgasm with penetrative sex.

Suggestion:

You aren't imagining things. This is most likely due to how the angle of your partner's penis relates to the position of penetration. This doesn't mean you should have to choose your partner based on the angle of his penis, but instead, you might need to find positions that work better for you and for him when you're having penetrative sex. If he's in a position where his pubic bone can provide direct stimulation to your clitoris, or where his penis will rub your clitoris directly as he thrusts, you might find you get enough stimulation to have an orgasm through penetration. You might also find that the angles just aren't quite going to provide enough direct stimulation no matter what positions you try. In this situation, using other methods of stimulation will help you to have orgasms.

The following positions are suggestions to help women figure out their needs. But as women get to know what works for them, I encourage them to keep track in their journals with the information for themselves. They might find that certain positions work better with certain partners, and not at all with other partners.

Positions to Delay Orgasms for Women

When it comes to penetrative sex for women, the vast majority of positions don't lead to orgasm. But many positions can bring a woman to the plateau stage and hold her there until both she and her partner are ready to orgasm.

Missionary position

In this position, there is very little stimulation directly on the clitoris, but the position can be quite pleasurable and can offer an opportunity to connect with your partner and sync your breathing. While it won't encourage orgasm, it will be a position that can raise your sexual response to a plateau level, and switching from missionary to a position that will increase the likelihood of orgasm can be easy to achieve.

Woman on top

In this position, women have control over the movement as well as the amount of pressure and stimulation to the clitoris. If you're looking to raise your sexual response but hold it steady, this position can offer that. Similar to the missionary position, woman on top allows you to change your position slightly to go from delaying orgasm to encouraging orgasm. Many women find that this position can also provide G-spot stimulation, but generally not enough to have a full G-spot orgasm.

From behind without additional stimulation

When your partner enters you from behind, this position can be very deep and can feel amazing, but without additional stimulation it won't provide any clitoral stimulation and won't result in a clitoral orgasm. The benefit of this position is that because your partner controls the depth and speed of penetration, you're free to enjoy the sensate focus and feel every movement he makes. It can definitely increase your sexual response without tipping you over the edge.

Man standing, woman lying down with legs up

With your partner thrusting into you from the side, he can again have the opportunity to vary the depth and speed of the penetration. Depending on the angle of his penis, he can use this position to hit your G-spot, provide different rhythms to tease you, and build toward orgasm without getting too close. This position is most easily achieved with the woman lying back on the bed or on a table as the man stands at the edge of the bed or table.

Sitting facing each other

This position offers great closeness, and the woman can have control over the speed and depth of penetration. By rocking her hips, she can also control the PC muscle, and by relaxing the PC muscle, she can have more time to build to orgasm slowly.

ENCOURAGING ORGASMS IN WOMEN

For many women, this is a much more difficult way to have an orgasm. Penetration alone can make orgasms difficult. In many of the positions that delay orgasms, slight variations can easily be turned into positions that encourage orgasm.

Positions that Encourage Orgasms for Women

Missionary elevated

By putting several pillows under the woman's bottom, orgasm will be more easily achieved. At this angle, her clitoris will be pressed against his pubic bone, and she'll be able to move her hips in rhythm with his on the pillows much more easily than on a hard surface. As she builds to orgasm, she may want to wrap her legs around him for extra pressure on her clitoris.

Woman on top variation

In this position, the woman can angle her body slightly, at a 45 degree angle to her partner, and use that angle to get more pressure on her clitoris. Instead of rising up and down on her partner, she can grind into him. This will give her the fullness in her vagina but also direct contact with his body on her clitoris.

The coital alignment technique

In this position, partners start in a missionary position. The male partner then moves his body up his partner's body. In this position, his erect penis is pointed more downward, so that the top of his penis is coming in direct contact with his partner's clitoris. As he thrusts, he moves his body down her body for the inward motion and up her body for the outward motion. This position can work for many couples, though some men find it causes an uncomfortable angle for their penis. I recommend trying this position a few times to see if it's something you and your partner enjoy. Generally, it's difficult to master the first time, so try not to abandon it too quickly unless it's uncomfortable to one or both of you.

From behind with a vibrator or manual stimulation

One of the greatest parts about rear entry is that the woman or man can have one or both hands free to stimulate the clitoris. In this position, there's easy access to the clitoris, and a vibrator or hand can be used to encourage orgasm. The additional G-spot stimulation will feel amazing as she gets closer to orgasm.

Scissors

By facing opposite directions and joining together their genitals as they split their legs, both partners can enjoy deep penetration and can use either the stimulation from the male partner's inner thigh, a vibrator, or hand to stimulate the clitoris. In this position, partners will have to communicate how close they're getting to orgasm, as it can be more difficult to negotiate. In this position, the woman must feel comfortable either asking her partner for stimulation or stimulating herself. The bonus is that if she stimulates herself, her partner might be incredibly turned on by the visual and by not being able to kiss her, and it's likely to send them both over the edge.

Man standing, woman lying down with legs up variation

As described above, when both partners are starting to feel their plateau come on stronger, the male partner is at the perfect angle to use his hand to rub his partner's clitoris or to use a vibrator on her. An added variation that can be very hot is to use some light bondage so the woman can't use her own hands and has to succumb to her partner's touches.

PC Muscle
and Orgasm

As a woman finds herself getting close to orgasm, squeezing and releasing her PC muscle can increase sensation, because it starts to involve all of the muscles around the genitals. By doing this, she can increase the sensation enough or relax enough to help match her partner's timing.

This might take some practice and the woman must have spent time doing her Kegel exercises to the point that flexing the PC muscle feels natural and comfortable to her.

Summary

Using sex positions is the final step in achieving simultaneous orgasms with your partner. By incorporating what you've learned in the previous chapters with the penetrative sex positions, you'll identify which positions work best for you and your partner together. Be prepared to try several different positions and to work together to determine your favorites. Don't be afraid to use manual stimulation or vibrators to help you have an orgasm. Not all of the positions mentioned in this chapter will work for every couple, and you might find that you need to make your own variations to have the best possible penetrative sex for your relationship.

HOMEWORK FOR MEN

Find what works: This part of the homework starts to become really fun for men! The goal of this activity is to try the positions mentioned in this chapter to identify what works to help men delay orgasm, and also what helps them achieve orgasm through penetrative sex. At this point, the goal is not to achieve simultaneous orgasm but to work on control and timing. Record your results to help you and your partner understand the best positions for you.

Try the delay: For this exercise, your goal is to get yourself as close to orgasm as you can and to try to use control to slow down your orgasm. Because it can be difficult to find the point of no return with penetrative sex, this might take a while to master. Try the stop-and-start method as well as the squeeze technique to see which is most comfortable for you and for your partner.

◉ HOMEWORK FOR WOMEN ◉

Find your position: Similar to the previous section, in this assignment the woman must find the position that works for her to delay and to encourage orgasm. Using the positions, the variations,
and the skills learned in the previous chapters, find the position
that's going to be comfortable to maintain, and also qualifies as
your go-to position for orgasm. This might take time and might
require your partner to use skills to delay his or her own orgasm.
Once you find your go-to positions, record them in your journal.

Work together: Now that you both have your positions, start
working together to find ways to combine the positions to synchronize your timing. At this point, you should be aware of your
sexual response cycle, your breathing, and which positions each
of you can reach orgasm in.

Make a sex menu: You now have the skills required to have
simultaneous orgasms, but you might need to make a plan that
will work for both of you to make your timing match. Add variations such as manual and oral sex and different positions. The fun
really starts when you can create multiple menus, or just go for it
and see what happens!

Goal Check-In: My past clients often focused their long-term goal
around having simultaneous orgasms with penetrative sex, and
achieving it was the culmination of their journey. If this is of inter-
est to you, consider using the short-term goals throughout the book
to build toward this destination.

ELEVEN

Troubleshooting

In this chapter, I cover some of the common issues that couples face as they try to achieve simultaneous orgasm together. Despite giving it a good effort, you might find that simultaneous orgasms are still not happening for you. Consider the following:

GIVING YOURSELF PERMISSION

It might sound a little crazy, but to get to where you want to be, you have to first give yourself permission to fail. Think of it this way: Bubba Watson had to miss a few cuts before he won the Masters. Scientists had to try more than one method before solving complex problems. Chefs had to burn a few dishes before opening a restaurant. You'll have to try a few times before you can achieve orgasm simultaneously, and that's OK. The goal isn't to make it happen immediately and accidentally, but to create a long-lasting and sustainable approach to consistent and reliable partnered orgasms.

SEX IS A SKILL

As much as we're all born with some innate level of a sex drive (the biological force that encourages us to be sexual), we aren't born with the knowledge of how to be good at sex. Sex is a learned or acquired skill, and learning how to do any skill takes time. The best way to do this is through practice—that's right, your homework is to have more sex with your partner.

Usually when I ask my clients to do this, I don't receive too many complaints.

By practicing with a partner, you have the opportunity to work on timing. By working together to understand how your bodies are working, you'll be able to find out how each of your sexual response cycles work, and how the timing can be matched.

Additionally, there are some days that no matter what partners do they're not going to be able to achieve orgasm together. We can chalk this up to stressors, hormones, moods, and various other external factors that are going to change sexual response cycles and emotions. Sometimes when this happens, the immediate response is to become upset or angry: after being successful, why isn't this working anymore? But if you can return to the idea that it's OK to fail, then the next time you try, you won't go into it with negative thoughts.

What's the most common cause of failing?

When people start thinking negative thoughts like "This will never happen!" they create a self-fulfilling prophecy. In many sexual issues, the main way to break the cycle is to avoid the negative response and start to think positively.

Your brain is the biggest sex organ you have, which can sometimes be a downside. Using too much of our brains, or going into a cognitive mode, prevents us from enjoying the emotional and experiential side of sex. As you progress through the activities in this book, you might find that you need to take some "time outs" to breathe. Too much focus on the simultaneous orgasms not happening is going to create issues that prevent you from relaxing and enjoying the orgasms you're having.

Our Timing Is Off

Syncing the timing for orgasms is definitely one of the most challenging aspects of this program. Some days it might come easily, and other days, it'll feel as if the two of you are on two different planets. Work together to communicate, and try communicating when you aren't in the throes of passion. Sit down over breakfast on a Saturday morning and talk about what the experience has been like for you.

Also, you should realize that sex doesn't have to result in simultaneous orgasms every time. It would be nice if that were the case, but it's not essential. Enjoying the sex you're having is much more important.

If you continuously find that you're missing the timing, but you're both having orgasms, you're on the right track! It might just take a bit more negotiating of the starting point or the positions you're using. Keep working on it and you'll definitely get there!

No-Go O

For some people, orgasms just don't seem to happen. There are a few things that could be going on.

Some known culprits in the O that won't go are antidepressant medications. Several medications get in the way of achieving orgasm; it's almost like they put a block into the sexual response cycle. Some people are able to get aroused, and even into the plateau phase, but they can't quite tip over the edge into orgasm. If you suspect that this could be a cause, check in with your health care professional. The good news is that there are several antidepressants on the market that are less likely to cause sexual function issues. There are also other ways to get around it, such as using an antihistamine to temporarily bypass the sexual issues and allow you to achieve orgasm.

Female Orgasms

For some women, achieving orgasms at all is an issue. I actually work with clients on this issue quite regularly, and it's difficult to summarize in just one chapter alone. If this is an issue that you or your partner is experiencing, you might decide to seek additional assistance from a sexologist or other clinical expert. Here are a few suggestions on how to achieve orgasms for women who have yet to experience an orgasm.

Try masturbation: Women sometimes fear or avoid masturbation because it feels wrong or they have negative associations with masturbation. Unfortunately, without knowing what it takes to have an orgasm alone, it becomes difficult to achieve an orgasm with a partner. Review the Self-Pleasuring chapter (page 72), and try a few of the techniques I've discussed. Try to make it your own, and relax and enjoy yourself!

Watch porn: Use the visual images to help stimulate you, turn you on, and push you from plateau to orgasm.

Use a vibrator: Many women find that the first time they're able to have an orgasm is through the use of a vibrator. Vibrators can give women that extra little push to get over the edge!

Breathing: In the Sexual Response Cycle (page 57) and Self-Pleasuring (page 72) chapters, I talked about using breathing to help get to climax. The method to getting to orgasm through breath is very common for women, and every woman experiences it differently. You may need to hold your breath, breathe more deeply, or breathe more quickly. Try out different combinations and see what works for you.

Muscle contractions and relaxations: Similar to breathing, some women contract and release muscles as they get closer to orgasm. Moving their legs closer together and tightening the muscles can send them into a sensation overload! Other women prefer to stay in a more relaxed position, and allow for a slower buildup to orgasm.

Relax! One of the most common issues is that women are so tense, so focused on getting that orgasm, that they can't let themselves enjoy their own pleasure and orgasm. They start creating their own self-fulfilling prophecy, thinking that they'll never reach orgasm, and guess what! With that mentality it sure is difficult to have an orgasm! Do what it takes to get into a state of relaxation. Enjoy the journey, and don't focus on the outcome.

Try different positions: Let your imagination be your guide! There are so many different positions that people can enjoy orgasms in. For some people, being in the bath or shower is a good place for them to experience orgasms, as it helps them relax and it feels like an intimate, personal experience. Others find that changing up their positions in bed can give them the change they need to boost them to orgasm. Try lying on your side, on your front, with the lights on, with the lights off, with your eyes open, or with your eyes closed.

Maintain clitoral contact! Constant stimulation will help achieve orgasms. For a lot of women, any change in the stimulation they're receiving can throw them off the orgasm train.

Kegel exercises: As I explained in the Anatomy and Physiology chapter (page 32), Kegels are an excellent way to maintain genital health and to feel more intense sensations. They also help women identify the different sensations they feel in their genitals, and help contract during orgasm. Follow the Kegel exercise plan and in no time you'll notice a significant difference in the awareness you have of your genitals!

Imagine yourself experiencing an orgasm: This is an exercise is also known as "Act as If." In this case, the woman is going to act as if she is experiencing an orgasm. Although this may sound like another way to say a woman is faking an orgasm, which I advise against in the Communication chapter (page 20), this exercise is not aimed at deceiving a partner; instead it's meant to encourage a positive response within the woman's own body. The woman imagines herself experiencing an orgasm, letting the body move, the sounds come out, and the pleasure waves surge through her body. It is usually recommended to first try this alone, while self-pleasuring. Many women get lost in the idea of the orgasm being or feeling a certain way. By doing the motions, and imagining having orgasms, it can connect the mental and physical and aid in getting over the edge from plateau to orgasm.

Move your hips! I once met with a yoga instructor who watched the way I moved and wondered how it was possible that I was so locked up through the hips. When I started thinking about this and applying it to the work that I do with clients I noticed that many women are locked through the pelvis. I now get them to incorporate some stretching and hip movement into the homework I give them. When they're able to access movement in their hips, orgasms are much easier for them to have. Incorporating some yoga stretches into your daily routine will help enhance and maintain hip flexibility. The positions I recommend to loosen the hips are taken from the teachings of Yin Yoga and can be found in *The Complete Guide to Yin Yoga* by Bernie Clark. The Frog, Happy Baby, Shoelace, Square, Squat, Dragon Fly, Swan, and various Dragon positions are all hip opening, and with continued practice will yield long-term benefits. As with any exercise, please consult a physician before proceeding. A professional yoga instructor will also be able to provide correct posturing instructions.

Women also find that they might have spontaneous hip movement, especially as they get closer to orgasm. Instead of being embarrassed, or trying to control it, give in to the movement and let your body do what it knows how to do!

Check in with a local sexologist: Look into a workshop for pre-orgasmic women or work with the sexologist to develop sessions for orgasm achievement!

FOR MEN

Erectile Issues

As men age, they tend to have less reliable and less firm erections. This is a normal part of getting older. Sometimes, though, loss of erectile function can indicate a more serious health condition, and you should have a physical examination by your health care practitioner.

If the issue persists and there are no health issues, one option is to discuss the situation with a sexuality specialist, such as a sexologist or sex therapist. A sexologist has been trained to support clients in achieving their goals through information and education, coaching, specific instructions, and counseling as needed. A sex therapist has been trained to use therapy to remove any psychological barriers to sexual success. Some will recommend looking into using a medication such as Viagra or Cialis, while others will use a nonmedical approach. The decision is up to the individual, but I do want to point out that using a medication alone will not help with sex drive or arousal, so if that's the main issue, I encourage people to follow up with the emotional and psychological factors in tandem with the physical factors.

In situations like this, I also encourage clients to aim to broaden their horizons; consider all sexual possibilities, rather than just penetrative sex. Men can still enjoy a lot of sexual pleasure through other types of sex. In this way, erectile issues can actually be seen as a blessing in disguise!

Early Ejaculation

Ejaculation prior to the desired time of ejaculation can be seen as a sexual issue for many men. This is a common concern to have and can be difficult to treat. The good news is that for many men, this issue diminishes significantly with age. The bad news is, it's difficult to wait for that to happen when you're trying to work toward simultaneous orgasms! Most men can last for about three to thirteen minutes with penetrative sex, which is about sixty thrusts.

The best way to start dealing with this issue is to get a good idea of what your sexual response is. By identifying what the feelings in the body are, you can become more aware of when you're getting closer to orgasm.

The next stage is to find a way that works for you to reduce the sensation, to go from almost going over the edge down to a manageable level. As described in the Positions for Men and Women chapter (page 114), several methods are available to reduce the sensations, so you just have to find the one that you're most comfortable with.

Some men find that they're so aroused by the time they get to have penetrative sex, they orgasm very soon after penetration. In this case, working on being calmer, breathing slowly, and focusing less on the final outcome will yield more positive results. If they do end up having an orgasm, they can wait out the refractory period and try again. As I mentioned in the Sexual Response Cycle chapter (page 57), the second orgasm can be delayed, because the penis can be less sensitive.

Another method to delay orgasm is to use condoms. Some men find that by using a condom, they have a slightly diminished sensation on their penis, and that might be just enough to help them have longer staying power.

Finally, practice, practice, practice! For men who get more experience, either by themselves or with a partner, they not only recognize the signs of getting closer, but also can build up more sexual stamina.

PORNGASMS?

One common issue is that people have seen or read porn and believe that it's easy to achieve simultaneous orgasms. News flash: They fake it in porn! They're actors, they don't always have orgasms, and very rarely do they have orgasms together. Unfortunately, the expectation set up by porn and other popular culture media for most people is not the reality. This creates expectations that only lead to frustration.

Porn has a place in many people's lives. Some people view it as a positive sexual enhancer, while others find it to be a horrible distraction from real life. However people look at it, there are positives and negatives to porn.

Porn can be a great way for couples to connect, get new ideas, increase their sexual desire, and boost their sexual response from plateau to climax.

When you watch or read porn, consider that these depictions of orgasm are akin to a fantasy. They can be pleasurable, but the realism is often absent from the way they show sex. When both you and your partner can acknowledge that what you've seen on the screen might not be reality, you can free yourself to experience your orgasms the way you experience them. Avoid negative self-talk and assumptions that something's "wrong" if you can't have an orgasm the way orgasms are presented in porn. Allowing yourself time and practice to understand your body and your partner's body will guide you together to the place you want to get to!

CONCLUSION

At this point, you have the knowledge and the skills you need to reach simultaneous orgasms! Now it's time to practice and develop the confidence you need to have simultaneous orgasms. Remember that failure is part of the process and part of the fun! The homework activities are there to help guide you, and you can always return to the homework at any time and can work with your partner if you need to go back a few steps.

Remember to enjoy the journey and not fight the process. As you become more aware of your own sexual response cycle, you'll become more prepared for the pleasure ahead of you. I wish you the best of luck as you continue on your sexual journey!

Glossary

69 An oral sex position that allows both partners to give and receive oral sex at the same time. Typically performed lying down, partners can lay side by side, or with one person on top and one underneath. This position can be very pleasurable for both partners and can result in simultaneous orgasm.

A-spot (Anterior Fornix Erogenous Zone) A newly discovered pleasure spot of females' bodies located deep in the vagina, on the front wall. Stimulation of this spot can result in very pleasurable sensations and also the rapid production of significant amounts of lubrication.

Clitoris The part of the female sexual anatomy whose sole responsibility is pleasure. The clitoris has over 8,000 nerve endings. The clitoral glans and hood are external and can be seen outside the body. The internal structure of the clitoris extends approximately 6 to 8 inches inside the body, running parallel to the labia.

G-spot (Graftenberg Spot) Also known as the urethral sponge, the G-spot is located on the anterior wall of the vagina, approximately 2 inches from the vagina's opening. Simulation of the G-spot can be intensely pleasurable and can result in G-spot orgasms.

Kegel Exercises A series of exercises that both females and males can do to strengthen the pelvic muscles, in particular the pubococcygeus (PC) muscle. Using Kegel exercises can increase the intensity of orgasms as well as keep the PC muscle toned and healthy.

Mutual Masturbation When couples use their hands to stimulate their genitals. They can stimulate their own genitals or their partner's.

Oral Sex When someone uses his or her mouth to stimulate their partner's genitals. This type of sex is often highly pleasurable for both male and female partners, and can be a turn-on for the person giving oral sex to their partner, as well. Many people use mutual oral sex to have simultaneous orgasms.

Penis The penis is part of the male sexual anatomy. It is responsible for three things: expelling urine, expelling ejaculate, and providing pleasure.

Sex Drive A person's motivation to engage in sexual activity with another person or persons. Sex drive can be spontaneous or can result from influences and other factors, such as intimacy, arousal, and emotional connection to a partner.

Sexual Response Cycle (SRC) The way human beings experience sexual feelings in their bodies. The SRC includes the physiological and emotional responses that a person has as they experience sexual arousal. The basic phases of the SRC are arousal, plateau, orgasm, and resolution.

Simultaneous Orgasm when partners are able to time their orgasms to happen at the same time. This is sometimes a spontaneous occurrence, but the majority of people do need to work with their partners to have orgasms together.

Vagina The vagina is the internal part of a female's sexual anatomy. Many people use the term "vagina" to describe the full female sexual anatomy, which is incorrect.

Vulva The proper anatomy term for the external sexual organs of a woman's body. It includes the inner and outer labia, clitoris, vaginal opening, and urethra. Some resources also include the pubic mons and the perineum as parts of the vulva.

References

BOOKS

The Big Book of Sex Toys: From Vibrators and Dildos to Swings and Slings—Playful and Kinky Bedside Accessories That Make Your Sex Life Amazing by Tristan Taormino (Beverly, MA: Quiver, 2009).

Moregasm: Babeland's Guide to Mind Blowing Sex by Claire Cavanah and Rachel Venning (New York: Avery, 2010).

The Guide to Getting It On by Paul Joannides (Waldport, OR: Goofy Foot Press, 2009).

The Hite Report: A National Study of Female Sexuality by Shere Hite (New York: Seven Stories Press, 2003).

For Yourself: The Fulfillment of Female Sexuality by Lonnie Barbach (New York: Signet, 2000).

Sex for One: The Joy of Selfloving by Betty Dodson (New York: Three Rivers Press, 1996).

Female Ejaculation and the G-Spot: Not Your Mother's Orgasm Book! by Deborah Sundahl (Alameda, CA: Hunter House, 2003).

The Good Vibrations Guide: The G-Spot by Cathy Winks (San Francisco: Down There Press, 1998)

The Ultimate Guide to Cunnilingus: How to Go Down on a Woman and Give Her Exquisite Pleasure 2nd edition by Violet Blue (Berkeley, CA: Cleis Press, 2010).

The Ultimate Guide to Fellatio: How to Go Down on a Man and Give Him Mind-Blowing Pleasure 2nd edition by Violet Blue (Berkeley, CA: Cleis Press, 2010).

The Ultimate Guide to Anal Sex for Women 2nd edition by Tristan Taormino (Berkeley, CA: Cleis Press, 2006).

139

The Ultimate Guide to Anal Sex for Men by Bill Brent (Berkeley, CA: Cleis Press, 2002).

Anal Pleasure and Health by Jack Morin (San Francisco: Down There Press, 1981).

The Complete Guide to Yin Yoga: The Philosophy and Practice of Yin Yoga by Bernie Clark (Ashland, OR: White Cloud Press, 2012).

SEX TOY STORES

United States

Good Vibrations

www.goodvibes.com

1620 Polk Street
San Francisco, CA 94109
415-345-0400

3219 Lakeshore Avenue
Oakland, CA 94610
510-788-2389

899 Mission Street
San Francisco, CA 94103
415-513-1635

308A (rear) Harvard Street
Brookline, MA 02446
617-264-4400

2504 San Pablo Avenue
Berkeley, CA 94702
510-841-8987

Babeland Toys

www.babeland.com

707 East Pike Street
Seattle, WA 98122
206-328-2914

94 Rivington Street
New York, NY 10002
212-375-1701

43 Mercer Street
New York, NY 10013
212-966-2120

462 Bergen Street
Brooklyn, NY 11217
718-638-3820

Early 2 Bed
www.early2bed.com
5232 North Sheridan Road
Chicago, IL 60640
866-585-2233

Adam and Eve
www.adamandeve.com
Online only.

Canada

Womyn's Ware
896 Commercial Drive
Vancouver, BC V5L 3Y5
604-254-2543
888-996-9273 (toll-free)
www.womynsware.com

Come as You Are
493 Queen Street West
Toronto, ON M5V 2B4
416-504-7934
888-504-7934 (toll-free)
www.comeasyouare.com

Good for Her
175 Harbord Street
Toronto, ON M5S 1H3
416-588-0900
877-588-0900 (toll-free)
www.goodforher.com

Acknowledgments

I've been very lucky to work with an amazing group of sexologists, sex educators, and sexual health professionals. Everyone I have worked with has influenced and aided me in this process. Thank you to those who have inspired me along the way. My husband, Justin, has been more supportive than any partner I could ever imagine. He is my biggest cheerleader and has provided the love and encouragement I needed to create this book. I love you, Justin!

I want to acknowledge my wonderful colleagues at Options for Sexual Health. Without them, I would not have the knowledge, compassion, or aspiration to educate that now have. I love having the opportunity to work with the group of like-minded individuals at Opt, and I appreciate all of you.

I truly have the most fantastic family in the whole world. They have supported me from day one and have always encouraged me to reach my goals. My parents, Ron and Dianne, have been the foundation on which my world has been built, and I am grateful to them every single day. My sister, Allanah, has been my comedic interlude, my entertainer, and my encouragement. Having a sister like her has given me the confidence I need to be who I am and to believe in myself. Bill and Elaine, you have probably been the most excited to see the finished product. I know it's not always easy to explain what your daughter-in-law does for work, but you have embraced it, and your pride in my career has meant the world to me!

About the Author

Dr. Ashleigh Turner-Corbeil is a clinical sexologist with a doctorate in human sexuality. In addition to seeing clients in her private practice, she is also a sexual health educator and provides educational workshops for adults. Through her education at the Institute for Advanced Study of Human Sexuality, Dr. Turner-Corbeil developed a broad range of understanding of sexual concerns and treatment options. Her goal is to help clients gain or return to the sexual functioning they desire. She lives and works in Vancouver, British Columbia.